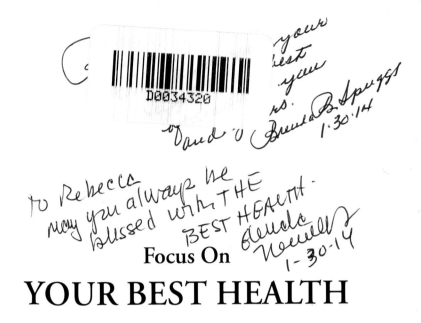

your
est
you
rs. Brenda B. Spriggs
1·30·14

and of

to Rebecca
may you always be
blessed with THE
BEST HEALTH.
Glenda
Newell
1-30-14

Focus On

YOUR BEST HEALTH

Glenda F. Newell, M.D.
Brenda B. Spriggs, M.D.

1ˢᵗ Printing

ISBN: 978-0-9791792-9-7

Please note that the internet websites listed as references and/or citations for further sources of information may have changed or become nonexistent between the time this book was written and the time it is being read.

Illustrations by Thaddeus Lavalais

Photography Credits
Glenda F. Newell, M.D. by Clifton Photography

Brenda B. Spriggs, M.D. by Mary Small Photography

A Note from the Authors

In order to assure confidentiality for our clients, friends, and family members who so graciously allowed us to share their medical experiences, all names and identifying characteristics have been changed or altered for the purpose of this publication.

dedications

The health and safety of my family is of the utmost importance to me. So, it is with unceasing gratitude and humility that I dedicate this book to my family: To my parents, Dr. Virginia K. Newell and the late George F. Newell, for endowing me with the best education, the grounding of family and unconditional love. To my sister, Dee Banks-Bright, M.D., for her gracious inspiration, matched with her refreshing sense of humor. To my older children, Tony and Regina, who have helped me to appreciate and enjoy a deeper, richer meaning of family. To my younger children, Brittany and Phillip, who constantly remind me — as they confidently follow their own paths, invigorated by the fundamental values of tenacity and determination — that my own perseverance was essential to completing this book. I am further grateful for their patience and tolerance when I was consumed with the extensive editing and phone calls. Above all, I dedicate this book to my husband, Bob, whom without his enduring love and unsparing support, this book would not have been possible. Finally, to my wonderful grandchildren and to those precious grandchildren yet to be born: I hope, someday, you will benefit from the concepts expressed herein…for your own best health.

Glenda

to my mother,
  Jewell,
    my inspiration

      to my children,
        Gabrielle and Zealous III,
          my joy

          to my life partner,
            Zealous,
              for encouraging me to
                pursue my own True North

                          BBS

Focus On
YOUR BEST HEALTH

Table of Contents

Preface

The American health care system is undergoing a seismic transformation, creating challenging barriers to staying healthy. Making medical decisions may be one of the most important tasks that we do, trumping financial and legal decisions – transactions we would never do without seeking help! Yet, today health care consumers are increasingly being asked to shoulder greater responsibility for making medical choices, and they are often simply not equipped to access or utilize the resources of today's health care environment. We have provided what we consider to be an insider's guide to making savvy medical choices. *Focus On YOUR BEST HEALTH* is an effort to guide patients through the complexities of receiving care – from the point of entry to the medical care system, to the doctor's office, to the hospital and beyond. It is a primer for those who want to develop simple, effective approaches to empowered healthcare – a smart, practical guide to patient survival in the medical trenches.

The clinical stories in *Focus On YOUR BEST HEALTH* demonstrate how enhanced medical knowledge, tactful coaching, polite assertiveness, and a better understanding of the healthcare system can have a positive impact on clinical outcomes. Our book is designed specifically to encourage patients to be intentional about medical needs and to help sharpen their ability to take charge of healthcare choices. Today's world of rapidly changing treatment information is often incomprehensible to the average patient, yet they are frequently asked to step into these rocky waters alone. The goal of *Focus On YOUR BEST HEALTH* is to optimize the healthcare experience, so patients can benefit from the advances of modern medicine.

Sadly, patients more often than not are themselves poorly informed and make choices in the absence of supportive coaches, such as relevant professionals, friends, and family members. It is our belief that those who provide structure during a medical crisis are frequently as important as the medical team that provides treatment. Throughout our professional careers in medicine, we also have found ourselves commiserating over the frequency with which family members or friends (patients themselves or supportive coaches) reached out to us for advice. We are well aware that advising friends and family has been, and most likely will continue to be, the norm for almost every physician. In our case, these situations have ranged from giving advice to a mother who wasn't sure of what to ask her child's pediatrician about a treatment, to a friend seeking reassurance and direction after receiving a diagnosis of breast cancer. Across friendship circles and family lines, many questions have recurred: *What type of subspecialist should I see? How do I tell my doctor I want a second opinion? What should I expect after this procedure? Should my condition be evaluated at a teaching hospital? How do I get my doctor to listen to me?* These occurrences were so frequent that they simply became a part of our routine life.

We have coached, advised, and advocated for family and friends on health-related matters since we were doctors-in-training. Most importantly, as mothers, wives, and trusted advisors, we are all too familiar with the frustration, fear, and angst triggered by illness. For all these reasons, we felt compelled to share our stories, perspectives, and expertise. We have practiced in many medical care delivery models and have an in-depth knowledge of the health care system: we know how it operates, what works, and what doesn't. Too often, we've witnessed the consequences of what doesn't work and the serious results that can occur when the system fails to meet patients' medical needs. In *Focus On YOUR BEST HEALTH*, we've drawn on our personal advocacy successes, as well as on our clinical experiences from academic settings, private practice, and community clinics, to offer practical and effective solutions to the common problems faced by health care consumers.

In revisiting these interventions, we identified common threads in the concerns expressed by friends and family members. These themes caused us to take a closer look at the root causes of the problems brought to us, then to monitor and assess any benefits that came from our interventions. A discovery quickly emerged. We identified three separate yet interrelated factors that were at the core of the issues raised by those seeking our help: *communication*, *navigation*, and *advocacy*. By identifying these three themes, we realized that our counseling had taken on a distinctive form. Through advocacy and coaching, we gave birth to *Focus On YOUR BEST HEALTH.*

As seasoned health care professionals, we have served as department chairs, medical directors, and presidents of physicians' organizations. Additionally, we have each served in volunteer roles, as directors of non-profit and for-profit boards, and held leadership positions in national organizations with major health care initiatives. To paraphrase, "We've looked at the medical scene from both sides now." Our involvement – locally, regionally, and nationally – has given us a broad and deeply nuanced appreciation of the role that quality health care plays in personal well-being. The vignettes we share represent a snapshot of our experiences and serve as real behind-the-scenes examples of the challenges and barriers facing health care consumers.

We know that access to medical care is often inextricably connected to costly health insurance and the byzantine rules that go along with it. We recognize the complexity and the burden of understanding insurance coverage, but we also know that having health insurance does not ensure quality health care. The insights presented in this book transcend any barriers that result from insurance matters. The subject of navigating insurance plans has been reserved for another publication and so will only be gently alluded to in this book.

Whether your medical encounters are routine or urgent, we believe that consumers must be educated about their health care needs, fully engaged in order to be active participants in medical decision-making, and empowered to take charge of their health. It is our hope that *Focus On YOUR BEST HEALTH* will serve as a survival tool to help you navigate your medical maze.

Focus On
YOUR BEST HEALTH

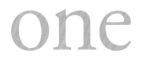

one

Health Care Communication Matters

"Communication works for those who work at it."

– John Powell

Try to imagine what your life would be like if you could not communicate your needs and desires. Think about planning a vacation, booking a contractor, or making a purchase. If you can't convey clearly what you want or expect from each task, you may not reach your expected destination with all of its amenities, obtain your preferred home remodeling plan, or guarantee your best purchase.

No one will die if you don't get the house remodeled the way you want or don't get a proper fit with that new pair of shoes, but when it comes to your health care, communication takes on more importance. In life-threatening situations, failure to communicate effectively can lead to poor clinical outcomes or even irreversible consequences. Yes, it's daunting to think about, but true. Clear, concise communication when addressing health matters is critical. And, in an ideal world, full engagement between a health care consumer and all members of the health care team is preferred.

As We See It...

As experienced physicians, we know how difficult it is for both patients and medical practitioners to be fully engaged during routine health care encounters. Every day, we see the reasons for this: time constraints, language barriers, and cultural differences, to name a few. These factors are major contributors to *communication barriers.* Our experiences have shown us that failure to recognize and overcome these barriers can have a negative impact on short - and long-term medical outcomes. Finding effective solutions to these barriers can result in positive outcomes, ranging from shorter hospital stays, to fewer infection complications, to improved functionality and a better quality of life.

If you are rushing to fill out a patient information form at the doctor's office, you might mistakenly enter the wrong information or skip a section of the intake form altogether. For example, you might omit your family history of breast cancer, which is significant information for screening schedules and treatment options. This problem could be avoided by requesting the required forms ahead of your visit, especially if you are a new patient. This will allow you the opportunity to inquire about important family history as well as gather your personal history for accuracy. It is also the responsibility of the doctor and the staff to make sure that questions are easily understood by a range of individuals with different cultural backgrounds and educational levels. In addition, the questions on the medical form should reflect the doctor's sensitivity to the level of medical knowledge in the general population.

The increasing diversity of our population dictates that health care systems and providers of medical services be more aware of the need to prevent language from becoming a barrier to care. If you don't speak the same language as your doctor, an appointment can become a wasted visit for you and lost time for the doctor. It can also result in inadequate medical information, which could lead to an inaccurate or missed diagnosis. Because the doctor relies on precise information in making decisions regarding your health care, the facts you share are crucial. When there are language barriers, you should notify the doctor's staff prior to your appointment. Ideally, arrangements for an interpreter should be easily accessible and instantly available. At larger medical and teaching facilities, this service is generally available and may include face-to-face interpreters, videoconferencing, or translation over the telephone. In our diverse society, it is the responsibility of all participants in the health care delivery system – doctors, patients, hospital personnel, and medical office staff – to be proactive in providing resources that will ensure clear, concise, and comprehensible communication.

"When the trust account is high, communication is easy, instant, and effective."

— Stephen R. Covey

Is Full Engagement Possible?

A meaningful relationship between a patient and a health care practitioner is formed in an environment where accurate information can be exchanged, where patient participation is expected and valued, and where there is a shared sense of openness and trust. This kind of relationship – *full engagement* – between patients and health care practitioners might sound like a pipe dream to some, but we believe it's achievable. Let's discuss how you can help make this a reality.

Let's Communicate

We hear the word *communication* a lot. But what does it really mean? The word is derived from the Latin *communis*, or "common." It means to share, impart, take part in, join, unite, or connect. In its simplest form, communication is a dynamic social interaction that involves the exchange of ideas between two or more people. Communication is one of the most important of all human behaviors. It allows us to ask for what we want, express our emotions, and relay important information to conduct our daily lives.

There may be special circumstances when patients are hearing impaired, which may require more attention and time to ensure successful two-way communication. What resources are used in these instances will depend on the severity of the impairment. Simply talking slower and allowing "teach-back" from the patient might benefit the parties involved, or a signing interpreter may be needed for more expert assistance. These modifications and resources are essential to enhance the understanding of shared medical information.

Why is communication so important to our health and the health of our loved ones?

As we've said, one of the most important places people communicate is in health care settings, where the stakes are high: poor communication can lead to missed or delayed diagnoses and inadequate or inappropriate medical care.

In a health care setting, effective communication is paramount. Both the health care practitioner and the patient will benefit from direct and honest sharing of information. This will result in a positive medical experience, will help to promote patient-doctor trust, and will lay the foundation for a viable partnership.

Breaking It Down...

There are four key components to effective communication: *verbal communication, non-verbal communication, active listening,* and *written/electronic communication.* We'll discuss the application of each of these components to health care settings later in this chapter, but in the meantime let's have a brief overview of them.

Verbal communication is pretty obvious: This is how we tell our stories and get our needs met through the spoken word. Every time we talk to our doctors about our medical condition, share concerns about our well-being, or discuss options for treatment, we are communicating. What you say about your health prompts the doctor to share medical knowledge, opinions, and recommendations with you. Or the doctor may ask you a series of health-related questions, to which you must respond factually and in detail. One of the best communication techniques that your doctor can use is to ask you open-ended questions. Instead of just asking you to respond with a simple *yes* or *no,* these kinds of questions allow you to fully express yourself. What exactly is an open-ended question? It is one that is designed to elicit from you, in your own words, more details and facts about your condition. Here are a few examples:

o "Could you tell me a little more about your discomfort?"

o "Will you please elaborate on how this pain limits you?"

o "Can you describe what has changed in your everyday routine as a result of this condition?"

o "What makes the problem better or worse?"

We know it is not always easy to speak up in a health care setting, whether you are seeing your regular primary care doctor or are being seen by a new doctor. But you should avoid falling into a pattern of answering questions with one word or a dismissive *"I don't know."* That is a conversation-ender, which will probably not contribute to additional sharing with your treating doctors or building a relationship with them.

Non-verbal communication is a way to get a message across without using words. Often, it amplifies what's being said: Sincere eye contact or certain facial expressions can show that the listener is approachable. Appropriate body language and the use of hand gestures may encourage better rapport. Non-verbal communication isn't always positive; it can also reflect disinterest, mistrust, or boredom. One very common complaint that we hear from people is that they feel rushed and uncomfortable when health care practitioners have one hand on the door while they are still talking. We call this "hand-on-door" syndrome.

Active listening is an important part of communication, which requires the participants to not only hear the words but understand the message. In a health care setting, the listener (whether doctor or patient) can give immediate feedback for clarification. These simple techniques will engage both parties. Remember, communication is a two-way street. If the listener does not understand the information being imparted, the communication is unproductive. To simply hear the spoken word is a passive exercise. The success of a communication exchange depends on both parties' ability to hear the spoken words, understand the message, and use purposeful listening techniques to enrich the experience.

"To listen well is as powerful a means of communication and influence as to talk well."

— Dr. John Marshall

We are well aware that in some instances patients report frequent interruptions from their doctor while they are sharing their medical concerns. It has also been reported that interruption dampens the desire of patients to continue sharing their medical history. This can lead to the doctor failing to obtain medical information that is critical to making a correct diagnosis. Such interruptions may appear to be rude, and they sometimes are. Nevertheless, it is important to be mindful of the reality of time constraints and pressures placed on doctors to see a certain volume of patients per day. If your office visit is fraught with interruptions, you might consider tactfully requesting that you be allowed to complete your story. If there are unpreventable time constraints, you should request another appointment. In summary, we cannot overstate the value of your role in providing pertinent, clear, concise, and accurate facts early on in the 15-minute appointment. Focus on what is important to you.

Electronic Communication in the health care setting is rapidly becoming the norm. Technology, however, can be a double-edged sword: In this overstressed world we all live in, it's great to have a fast, efficient way to share information. However, the transition from paper to an electronic medical record (EMR) system is both time-consuming and distracting for the medical doctor, whether in a hospital or an out-patient setting. We frequently hear from people that they are upset about the lack of eye contact between them and health care practitioners, who may be inputting data into a computer instead of engaging them in dialogue. For some medical staff and physicians, the learning curve for EMR proficiency is steeper than for others. The process for data entry is time-consuming and cumbersome, and in many instances conflicts with how doctors were trained to document medical information. As a result, this technology can add more stress, workload, and confusion to an already complex system. Continual improvement and upgrading of EMR software to meet the needs of medical advances will continue to challenge medical practitioners.

So, how do you participate in this electronic process? The common practice now is to provide you with a medical summary from the EMR at the end of your visit. This may include important information, such as your diagnosis, medications, and treatment plan. It is up to you, the patient, to read these documents thoroughly, understand the information presented, and correct any errors regarding your history and diagnosis. This is your permanent record.

Accessing Your EMR

Your ability to access your electronic medical records has significant advantages and disadvantages:

o   One advantage is that you have ready access to some of the laboratory results contained in your record and the ability to log in from home or at your workplace. This information can also be shared with family members as well as subspecialists if you have been referred to one and there is a delay in the transfer of your hard-copy medical records.

o   One disadvantage is that, on occasion, the system can break down completely, requiring you to produce written materials that would ordinarily be accessible electronically. This can range from upcoming appointments and pending referrals to current medications and dosages prescribed. This is where *Your Personal Health Record (YPHR)* comes into play (as will be discussed later in this chapter).

Electronic Medical Records: Not A Panacea

While electronic medical records are being universally adopted as the gold standard for medical documentation, they continue to be a challenge. The disadvantages of EMRs are gradually being recognized. For example, hospitals and other health care facilities often use different software programs that are incompatible with each other, which defeats one of the primary goals of hassle-free, system-wide access to patient health records. Software incompatibility often requires health care practitioners and ancillary health care workers to call and/or fax important medical documentation, which defeats the whole point of the paperless process.

Another hurdle impeding a smooth transition to this perceived panacea is that EMR formats are not compatible with how veteran health care practitioners were trained to document medical information.

In the long run, health care consumers will be the ones most impacted negatively by the implementation of electronic medical records. How?

o   Inadequate and insufficient technical training for EMR implementation can result in frustration and wasted time for the doctor, causing a distraction from the task at hand.

o Insufficient face-to-face patient-doctor interaction can lead to patient dissatisfaction.

o The focus on electronic inputting detracts from effective sharing of medical information and engagement by both parties.

These issues are likely to worsen as the insured patient population and doctor shortage increase. The time and effort that health practitioners devote to mastering electronic medical records decreases their clinical productivity and, therefore, decreases patient access to them. It's a domino effect!

So, let's take a look at some of the positive aspects of this system. A survey of our colleagues reveals some attractive and practical aspects of electronic medical records:

o With a few clicks and a push of a button, prescriptions can be quickly sent electronically to a pharmacy (which also decreases errors and/or handwriting issues).

o Electronic medical records are capable of creating medical visit summaries for patients.

o Electronic communication among medical staff members ensures legible documentation of orders, patient progress, and clinical management plans.

o These systems provide ready and quick access to all charts online (which saves time searching for patient charts).

o Direct access by both doctors and patients to lab tests and x-ray results allows for efficient and timely clinical decision-making.

The time factor is critical in medical settings, since doctors and other health care practitioners are up against the clock when they see patients. Critical data entry is challenging and likely to get worse with increasing patient loads.

You, the health care consumer, must demand that your medical encounters remain personal. Face-to-face encounters are the mainstay for meaningful patient-doctor interactions, providing opportunities for relationship enhancement. They are also valuable because they contribute to doctors' in-depth understanding of their patients.

When it comes to electronic and written communications, both the patient and the health care practitioner should aim to be concise and clear. Patients must be accurate in relating their medical history and describing symptoms. Health care practitioners should clearly explain the need for laboratory tests, x-rays, and other procedures. And both parties should employ active listening to avoid any misinterpretations created by oral communications.

Your First Encounter with Your Doctor

Preparation for meetings is something we do all the time. We prepare for meetings with our accountants, our attorneys, and our children's teachers. And when we meet them, we often think of ourselves as interviewing them: Are they competent to handle our money? Can they help us resolve our legal issues? Are they qualified to teach our children? Even if it's a first encounter, we come to them with the desire to share information, get answers to our questions, and, hopefully, leave with confidence in their abilities.

Why not take the same approach with your doctors? You are there to interview them, share information, document your health status, and have baseline testing performed. This is no small matter. The quality of the information that you bring – your personal medical history and family history – will be reflected in your permanent medical record, giving your physician important facts to understand you and your health. With enough data, you can give your doctor ample opportunity to formulate the best working diagnosis and treatment plan. This is a crucial step, since it directly impacts your ongoing medical management, your preventive care screening and monitoring, and ultimately your clinical outcomes and future well-being.

Looking for a Doctor? Is This a Fit?

Your choice of a doctor should be based on a number of factors. While health care consumers increasingly rely on the internet as a source of background information on doctors, there are some questions that we feel you should ask in a face-to-face encounter. Remember, you are interviewing the doctor to determine if this is the right fit for you. What kind of questions would you want to ask if you were meeting a primary care doctor for the first time, hoping to establish a relationship? What preparations should you make before your visit? What expectations are appropriate? From the doctor? From the visit?

The next questions are some that you should consider when choosing a doctor. The answers may come from various sources during your due diligence and should reassure you that your choice of a doctor will meet or exceed your medical needs.

Questions for Doctors:

- o Where was your medical school education and residency training?
- o What is your position on preventive care, and how does it fit into your medical management?
- o How open are you to alternative forms of treatment?
- o What provisions do you have for urgent or same-day medical care?

o Are you available for evening or weekend appointments?

o What are your hospital affiliations?

o Are you affiliated with preferred subspecialists or centers of excellence?

While we know that there are many additional questions you might want to ask, these are just a few that we think are important to help you organize your thoughts for that first visit. If the doctor meets your expectations, this may be a fit!

Being Interviewed by Your Doctor

There are a few ground rules that we feel your doctor should follow when interviewing you. The doctor should:

o Ask pertinent questions regarding your medical condition or complaint.

o Comment appropriately as you relate your personal history.

o Show empathy when appropriate.

o Ask open-ended questions to allow you to elaborate.

o Allow you to repeat your understanding of your condition and treatment plan.

o Use plain English rather than medical jargon.

o   Make interpreter services available when necessary.

o   Recommend a follow-up visit if all issues cannot be addressed.

Remember, because of limited time available for your visit, it is important that you share the most relevant and pressing facts about your problem within the first few minutes of the visit.

If this is a first visit with a new doctor, and you have a specific medical complaint, tell your medical story and describe your symptoms clearly to ensure the most accurate diagnosis. First of all, you must tell the doctor what brought you to the office and specifically what your symptoms are. If you are not critically ill and can speak, you should be prepared to answer questions such as:

o   What is your primary concern today?

o   Do you have pain, weakness, or fever?

o   Do you have chest pain or breathing problems?

o   How long has this been a problem?

o   Have you been treated for a problem like this before?

o   When was the last time you were able to function normally?

We recommend writing down your medical concerns, symptoms, and questions in advance and bringing them with you to your appointment. Here are our top 15 questions for you to ask at the end of your visit, depending on the circumstances:

1. What is my diagnosis/problem?
2. Do I need more testing for my problem?
3. What can I expect from the testing?
4. Can my condition be treated?
5. How will my condition be treated?
6. Will I need medication?
7. Do I have to take it all the time?
8. Should I see a specialist?
9. Are there other alternative methods of treatment available to me?
10. Will this condition affect my usual routine?
11. Can I exercise?
12. Can I travel?
13. What should I change in my everyday life?
14. Are the labs and medications covered by my health insurance?
15. How soon should I expect to get better?

Now that you've had your first visit, you are reflecting on your experience at home. Here are a few key questions you might ask yourself to determine if your needs were met:

Your Medical Evaluation

o   Were you allowed time to adequately relate your medical problem?

o   Did you feel that the doctor was "hearing" you?

o   Did the doctor examine you?

Testing and Procedures

o   Were the diagnostic tests explained clearly?

o   Were your questions about the rationale and purpose of the testing answered?

o   Did you understand the impact of the testing on your future treatment?

o   Were possible side effects and risks discussed?

o   Did you understand what you needed to do to prepare for the testing?

Even when you have prepared for your medical visit and have made efforts to seek clarification, things aren't always smooth sailing. Here's an example of what can happen when important information isn't clearly communicated or documented.

From Our Case Files...

R.S. *(not her real initials) is a 58-year-old female who has been treated for high blood pressure over a five-year period. During that time, she has taken two medications to treat her high blood pressure, one of which is a diuretic (water pill). At a recent weekend health fair at her church, her blood pressure was noted to be very high (160/96). The patient was alarmed and reported it to her doctor on her regular Monday morning visit. The patient was a little anxious, and her blood pressure at this visit was 130/86, which was only slightly higher than normal. The doctor then discussed his concerns and informed the patient that if she continued to have elevated blood pressure, he might have to add a third medication. He reviewed her medications and her dosing schedule, and wanted to make sure that R.S. was taking the medications as prescribed. R.S. informed him that if she needed another medication, she would take it, but if it caused her to go to the bathroom any more than the current medication did, she would have to take a "medicine holiday" on Sundays.*

What is going on here? R.S. has been head usher at her church for ten years. Her current doctor of six years diagnosed her high blood pressure. What was missing in her intake history? R.S. probably was not compliant with her medications, because she now runs to the bathroom more frequently. She may not have shared her responsibility as a church usher with her doctor. In addition, the doctor never asked directly if she took her medications every day, but instead asked if she took her medications as prescribed. Regardless of the reasons, this problem was a result of ineffective communication by both patient and doctor.

The underlying issue in R.S.'s case was that she didn't take her diuretic blood pressure medicine daily. Many patients are reluctant to tell their doctor that they have not followed instructions regarding medications, and some do not understand why they need to take the medications as prescribed. Unless a catastrophic event occurs, most instances of patient non-compliance with medication go unnoticed. Why? Patients are hesitant to reveal this because they fear being judged or reprimanded by the doctor. There is still that sense of the doctor as an authority figure for many patients, which can pose a real communication barrier.

Social, Cultural, and Religious Background: It may seem irrelevant to share your social history, culture, and religious practices when engaging with your health care practitioner, but this information is important to discuss. It is a common oversight by patients and health care practitioners to discuss daily activities and routine habits; yet these influence our overall health and well-being. Certain religious practices require fasting for long hours, which obviously can affect certain patients with diseases such as diabetes. In fact, some patients may simply stop taking their required morning medications in order to comply with their cultural or religious practices. Therefore, it is important for you to share your customs and practices and for the doctor to inquire about such cultural matters. Communication and exchange of this type of information not only gives your doctors a better understanding of your condition, but will allow them to manage your care more efficiently.

As a regular practice, we believe that health care practitioners should ask their patients if they are taking their medicines every day – especially when the medicine is not providing the expected results. That discussion may lead to new solutions and options for your medical management. Moreover, there are many different medications to treat high blood pressure. It's easy to offer a substitute medication or prescribe additional medications to the treatment regime in an effort to control the blood pressure. However, if your doctor does not know whether you are taking the original medications consistently, he or she may overprescribe medications for you, which can lead to serious side effects. All this can be avoided with better communication.

We know that failure to follow doctors' medication recommendations can be a result of many factors, such as your lack of trust. You may also have family members or friends who had bad or difficult medical experiences, or you just do not want to take medicines all the time. In addition, you may experience annoying side effects, and are either hesitant to tell the doctor or you simply dismiss these symptoms as being unrelated to the medication.

Health care professionals can do better by explaining potential side effects to you and inviting you to report *any* differences in your well-being. You can do better, too. Both parties must do their part to value and optimize the exchange of pertinent medical information. Effective communication will go a long way to ensure your adherence and improve your medical experience.

In our current hurried health care system, with doctors having limited time, it is not surprising that we are witnessing more and more non-compliance by patients. There is little time for teach-back, which could solve some of the problems, especially those involving medication dosing. You should ask what the dosing schedule should be and if stopping the medication or missing doses could present a serious problem. It is your right to know, and it is your responsibility to comply with all medication recommendations.

When we look at the doctor-patient encounter in general, we see critical communication opportunities for the doctor to achieve better patient satisfaction and, ultimately, to improve compliance. Thiedke (2007) cites five ways that doctors can attain patient satisfaction:

o Demonstrate and communicate empathy when appropriate.

o Give patients the time and opportunity to tell their story.

o Explain medical information and instructions clearly.

o Encourage patients to express their expectations, ideas and concerns.

o Acknowledge the importance of patients' social lives.

This brings us back to our first example, the case of R.S. Her doctor was not aware of her church duties as an usher. Also, R.S. did not know that taking a "medicine holiday" could cause her serious problems.

What About Looking At the Whole Patient?

The term *holistic health* gets tossed around a lot, so you may hear it used by some practitioners. What exactly is it, and how does it relate to you? The American Holistic Association (2012) defines holistic health as "the conscious pursuit of the highest level of functioning and balance of the physical, environmental, mental, emotional, social, and spiritual aspects of human experience, resulting in a dynamic state of being fully alive."

This sounds like a great state of health for us all, but most health care practitioners are not trained to focus on this all-encompassing approach to patient care. The emergence of integrative medicine and patient-centered care provides a platform on which the *whole* patient is considered, along with the social and environmental factors that influence the patient's well-being. This patient-centered approach uses therapeutic interventions from both traditional and alternative medicine (Maizes, Rakel, & Niemiec, 2009).

Unfortunately, the reality of the practice of medicine today is that health care practitioners are constrained by time, resources, and the economics of reimbursement for services. Non-traditional health options are often not explored by most practitioners, especially those who have been in practice for more than twenty years. This is due to a number of factors, including the lack of specific insight and training in the discipline, fear of embracing "unproven" remedies, and lack of knowledge of scientific research that supports alternative modes of treatment.

From a health and wellness perspective, we can

still work toward embracing the concept of a holistic approach, addressing social, cultural, and emotional influences, and considering how alternative therapeutics can influence a patient's treatment and compliance.

The Ask Me 3™ *Program*

Achieving effective communication does not have to be complicated. A unique but simplistic concept to ensure better communication and patient understanding of medical conditions and instructions is the Ask Me 3™ program. We know that improved understanding through better communication leads to improved patient compliance and ultimately better health outcomes. This program encourages patients to understand the answers to three questions (Ask Me 3™, 2011):

1. What is my main problem?
2. What do I need to do?
3. Why is it important for me to do this?

Utilizing these three questions during the medical encounter will help patients understand what their problem is, what they need to do, and why it is important to follow all their doctor's instructions. This includes laboratory requests, medication schedules, and any other prescribed orders or recommendations.

When miscommunication occurs, no one person is to blame. Both patient and practitioner are responsible for ensuring that health information is fully shared. An example of missed doctor-patient communication occurs when a patient fails to ask, or a doctor fails to explain, the value and rationale of tests or x-rays ordered to evaluate medical problems. Testing provides critical information to the doctor, but you must be confident that the testing is necessary and relevant for your condition.

The more information candidly exchanged between doctor and patient, the more mutual confidence and trust there will be. Trust is personal and must be developed over time. Being engaged in the medical process by asking questions is an excellent first step.

Effective Medical Team Communication Prevents Medical Errors!

Medical errors usually happen when important patient information and instructions are inaccurate, missing, misinterpreted, or inadvertently dismissed as unimportant. These errors can be written, spoken, or electronic. Any miscommunication, misinterpretation, or failure to communicate important lab data or clinical findings can have untoward and sometimes very serious consequences. That is why all clinical information must be concise and accurate at all times, and concerns or questions regarding intent or accuracy of a communication must be addressed promptly.

When we consider communication in the health care setting, the first thing that comes to mind is doctor-patient communication, and specifically the patient interview. But what about communication among health care personnel themselves? Health care probably has one of the greatest "hand-offs" of consumers of any other industry. In the hospital setting in particular, there are work shifts for nurses and doctors, and any miscommunication during the transfer of care, whether it is a shift change or a change of facilities, can have serious consequences. Because of potential medical errors, reporting on a patient's condition must be done shift-to-shift and should include the input of all members of the team who care for a particular patient. This critical hand-off requires time and commitment from the entire medical team, who are often faced with reduced staffing.

OOPS!

So, what are the consequences of miscommunication? These can be minor or major, but since patient safety should always be the top priority, they are *all* important. Research has shown that medical errors are directly related to poor communication between doctor and patient or between doctors, nurses, and other medical personnel. According to JCAHO (Joint Commission on Accreditation of Healthcare Organizations), 65 percent of all unexpected occurrences leading to death or other serious physical or mental injury, occurring between 1995 and 2004, were caused by communication problems. In 2005, a JCAHO study revealed that 70 percent of medical errors leading to death or serious injury were caused by communication breakdown, 50 percent of which occurred during patient hand-offs (Runy, 2008).

Medical errors do not have to be as dramatic as surgical mishaps, but anything that happens with the potential to adversely affect a patient is a medical error. These can be prescription errors (wrong drug, wrong dose, wrong dosing schedule, medication interactions) that can result from lack of knowledge on the part of the patient, doctor, caregiver, or pharmacy. These potential life-threatening errors require you to understand all medication instructions that can affect your well-being or that of your loved ones.

When Things Go Wrong...

A typical encounter with your doctor usually consists of history taking and physical examination, followed by ordering laboratory tests as needed. Such requests can include a complete blood count, cholesterol screening, and a urine test. This seems straightforward, right? Not always. There are cases in which tests ordered by the doctor are inadvertently omitted during processing in the laboratory. Mistakes made during the transcription or execution of written or electronic communications relating to laboratory testing can lead to time-consuming corrections. For example, the doctor may have to repeat orders and may require patients to return to the lab for the proper testing to be done. This can be costly because of charges generated for each visit, not to mention the added factor of patient inconvenience. And it can pose a danger to the health of the patient if a diagnosis is missed or treatment is delayed due to lack of lab results.

Let's take a look at a case in which a laboratory transcription oversight could have resulted in serious consequences.

From Our Case Files...

W.H., a 55-year-old financial advisor, was seen by his primary care physician for chills, fever, and the possibility of a urinary tract infection. His primary care doctor ordered routine lab tests and blood cultures. The technician transferred the orders from the primary care doctor's electronic request onto labels for the phlebotomist (the person who draws blood). Prior to the blood draw, W.H.'s wife, a medical doctor, knowing that her husband was a difficult "stick" (had veins that were hard to draw blood from), asked the phlebotomist if he had obtained enough blood for the requested blood cultures. "Blood cultures?!" the phlebotomist exclaimed. "No blood cultures were ordered!" Much to the dismay of W.H., his wife, and the phlebotomist, the technician had failed to transcribe that particular lab test when making the labels. Because the correct tests were not performed, a potential diagnosis and cure could have been overlooked.

What is the lesson here? This is an example of failed communication between the doctor and the technician, involving electronic transmission of tests ordered. People assume that electronic communication is 100 percent accurate and fail-safe. But, as you can see from this scenario, that is not the case. Machines cannot replace humans. We must still rely on human beings to understand, interpret, and transcribe medical requests appropriately. This type of failed communication can result in missed diagnoses, inappropriate treatment, and dire medical outcomes. If the primary care doctor had assumed that the requested lab work had been done, and if antibiotics had been started immediately following the lab visit, this would have resulted in a missed opportunity to determine whether an infection was in W.H.'s bloodstream.

Why is this important? Conditions such as urinary tract infections and pneumonia, which have the potential to reach the bloodstream, may require hospitalization and should be diagnosed and treated as quickly as possible. If untreated, such infections can result in major complications, including death.

The point about this breakdown in communication is clear. However, we should also look at this situation as an indication of how busy and challenged many hospital staff can be. Also, increased workloads, multitasking, and staff shortages contribute to distractions for hospital personnel and can interfere with the proper execution of doctors' medical orders.

How many patients actually pay attention to what lab tests are ordered? Imagine what the outcome could have been if W.H. had not been accompanied by his wife, a medical professional. If this oversight and potential breech of procedure can be made under these circumstances, imagine the exposure that patients without advocates can have.

This case is an example of how medical errors can occur in health care settings. The Institute of Medicine (1999) has defined medical errors as the "failure of a planned action to be completed as intended or the use of a wrong plan to achieve an aim." We know that the majority of medical errors are preventable. We also know that more than 98,000 patients die each year as a result of such errors. If we look at the reasons why medical errors occur, we will find poor oral and written communication at the top of the list. These occurrences are not isolated to any particular type of medical encounter or to any medical specialty. They happen among health care personnel and professionals at every level of the health care delivery system. That's why we feel so strongly about effective communication, whether spoken or written.

What role can *you* play in reducing medical errors when it comes to your health?

Be aware of what testing is being ordered by your doctor, and ask why the test is being done. Your questions should include:

o Will only blood be required?
o Do I have to give a urine sample?
o Should I be fasting (nothing by mouth for 12 hours) before testing?
o Is it advisable to draw the blood if I have eaten?
o If blood cultures are indicated, should the new medicine prescribed be taken before the blood is drawn?

These simple questions will not totally prevent laboratory testing errors, but should make you aware, at a very basic level, of what is needed from you to complete the doctor's orders. We also know that most instructions are given to you in a written form by the doctor, with the expectation that you will read them. For example, if you have read and have been told that a urine sample is needed, you are not likely to leave the testing laboratory without providing a urine specimen, which often happens. However, most people in our rushed society do not take the required time to read and digest the written communication.

Your Personal Health Record

Another important and highly valuable form of written communication is *Your Personal Health Record (YPHR)*. This useful document should be accessible to you, your family, or your caregiver at all times. We strongly urge you to have a personal health record with the following information: medical conditions, medications, allergies, surgeries, hospitalizations, and immunizations. The information in this format can be especially helpful in the emergency room or when you are on vacation. *Your Personal Health Record* will be invaluable, giving the treating doctors a snapshot of your medical history. *(See Appendix I for our recommended version of Your Personal Health Record.)*

We recommend including the following information for *Your Personal Health Record:*

o   Past and present medical disorders.

o   Past and present medications, including prescriptions, over-the-counter drugs, and dietary herbal supplements.

o   Allergies or adverse reactions to foods or medications.

o   Dates of routine preventive care procedures,

including eye exams, colonoscopies, mammography exams, etc.

o Immunizations.

o Family history.

o Previous hospitalizations and surgeries.

o Emergency contacts.

o Health insurance information.

This information can be written on a card, saved on a Universal Serial Bus (USB) memory stick, or placed on a website that specializes in setting up your personal health record. The contents of this personal health record can be shared with family members, health care practitioners, and emergency room doctors, as needed. If your doctor is set up for electronic medical records, you may be able to access your recent lab and x-ray results. If you have your most recent lab and x-ray test results in your possession, and can make them available to a radiologist or any other subspecialist, this might help you to get your appointment scheduled sooner.

"What you do speaks so loud that I cannot hear what you say."

— Ralph Waldo Emerson

More on Non-Verbal Communication and Active Listening

Communication is a two-way street, involving the person delivering or sharing the information and the person receiving the information. Studies show that a surprising 85 percent of all human communication is expressed by body language and other non-verbal means. Therefore, it is critical to recognize both the positive and negative impacts of this form of communication.

Positive non-verbal communication and active listening are essential for quality patient-doctor interactions. This kind of communication sets the tone for each party to feel at ease to ask questions, express opinions, exchange information, and fully understand what the other person is trying to communicate. Positive non-verbal communication and active listening also foster trust and allow doctors the maximum opportunity to get accurate medical information.

A major reason why patients switch doctors is their perception that they are not being heard. They feel that their health care practitioner is simply not "hearing" them. We know that both doctor and patient need to communicate a baseline of facts. But it's not just about the data. A patient wants to feel that the practitioner is a partner in the health care process. If treating practitioners are actively listening and can acknowledge, in some way, that they are receptive to the fears, anxieties, and concerns of their patients, this is a good start to building trust and allowing patients to feel that they are being heard.

Positive Non-Verbal Communication Techniques Used by Doctors

As a patient, you should be aware of a few very simple non-verbal communication techniques that some doctors use to create an environment of trust, to actively listen, and to build a solid doctor-patient relationship:

o   They establish and maintain eye contact.

o   They sit or stand at the same level as the patient.

o   They use appropriate head nodding to acknowledge information.

o   They lean forward to indicate engagement.

Let's examine the case of a seasoned corporate psychologist who was concerned and alarmed at the negative non-verbal communication exhibited by her doctor. This behavior interfered with her ability to get timely and crucial information from her doctor that she needed to make an important health care decision.

From Our Case Files...

W.T., a 46-year-old practicing psychologist, had a recent mammogram that revealed an abnormality requiring further investigation. A week later, she was seen by a breast specialist, but was so troubled by the doctor's behavior and was so anxious about her own condition that she could not fully comprehend the recommendations from the specialist. Because of her confusion, W.T. decided to make another appointment with the specialist as soon as possible, hoping that a second visit would give her a better understanding of her condition and the appropriate next steps. When her spouse asked about her visit, W.T. informed him that the specialist never made eye contact with her, appeared rushed, and answered his cell phone twice during the visit. The doctor also appeared annoyed when W.T. became emotional while attempting to relate her history. W.T. asked her spouse if he would accompany her to her next visit, and he agreed. Upon W.T.'s return visit to the breast specialist, the doctor entered the room, greeted the patient and her spouse, extended his hand to the patient, and sat down to review the highlights of the previous visit. He reviewed his recommendations and allowed the patient to ask questions. He also discussed treatment options and an appropriate time frame for next steps. Before W.T. left the office, the doctor asked her to repeat the options (teach-back) to be certain of her understanding. Because of this surprising and refreshing approach on the part of the doctor this time around, the patient was less anxious and was able to articulate her concerns more clearly. The doctor expressed a genuine interest in W.T.'s medical concerns and was clear and concise regarding what needed to be done. The spouse sat in, but did not actually participate in the dialogue.

What is the lesson here? The initial encounter was dreadfully unsuccessful for a number of reasons, including negative non-verbal communication, time constraints, the patient's fears, and the absence of an environment where the patient felt safe and comfortable to share her medical concerns. The doctor's perceived lack of empathy and his obvious distractions caused W.T. to feel that things were spiraling out of control. She literally could not hear or absorb what the doctor was saying because of the negative non-verbal communication. W.T. left her initial visit without the information she desperately needed. We know that everyone on occasion has a bad day, so that may explain the doctor's behavior and responses to the patient at the time of the initial visit. But when a doctor is faced with the task of explaining information about a dreaded disease, it is important for the doctor to waltz delicately.

Medical settings are typically not warm and inviting places. When patients are fearful or compromised physically or emotionally, an empathetic ear makes the situation bearable. We feel that whenever you feel uncomfortable in a medical appointment, you should make arrangements for someone to accompany you to your future visits. This could be a colleague, friend, family member, or anyone else who might serve as an advocate for you.

Because of the increasing demands on doctors, patients must be even more vigilant than ever in recognizing any shortcomings that might adversely affect their patient-doctor encounters. You, the patient, should be able to voice your concerns and expectations without fear of judgment or rejection. The presence of the spouse at the second encounter gave W.T. the emotional support she needed. He was also a silent advocate, which can be invaluable in a medical setting.

How Non-Verbal Communication Can Help or Hinder

The case of W.T. is a classic example of how non-verbal communication can hinder the patient-doctor encounter. There are various examples of non-verbal communication that can have a negative impact. Anxiety in one's voice or tension in the shoulders influence how your message is received. Hand and arm gestures can also impede your positive engagement in a medical setting. However, non-verbal communication goes both ways. It can be harmful or helpful to the relationship.

Here are a few examples of non-verbal communication involving patient and doctor:

Negative Non-Verbal Communications	Doctor	Patient
Failure to Establish Eye Contact	X	X
Multi-tasking (phone, interruptions)	X	X
"Hand-on-door" Syndrome Rush to Exit	X	
Avoiding Answering Direct Questions	X	X
Folding of Arms (Implying Unavailability)	X	X
Use of Stop Sign Gesture	X	X
Inattentiveness Due to Time Constraints	X	X
Distraction Due to Family Needs/Stress	X	X
Pointing Finger While Giving Instructions	X	
Rigid Focus on Data Entry (EMR)	X	

We encourage you to be more aware of how you are communicating non-verbally with your doctor and realize the importance of positive engagement. If your doctor routinely uses the gestures that we previously have noted, you may need to think about how he or she makes you feel.

Whether it is the doctor or the patient who is communicating negatively, that will affect how your medical needs are addressed. If the practitioner is conducting a patient interview or seeking medical information in an urgent situation, the medical encounter will definitely be enhanced by a genuine display of concern and body language that invites dialogue and encourages engagement.

We must not overlook the fact that there are positive postures and hand gestures that the doctor can make, which can encourage sharing, trust, and engagement on the part of the patient. Some of these are:

o   Greeting the patient with a genuine handshake.

o   Leaning forward with interest.

o   Placing a hand on the patient's shoulder if comfort is deemed necessary and appropriate.

o   Listening with a posture of thoughtfulness and curiosity.

o   Nodding and/or smiling to indicate agreement, understanding, or approval.

o   Open hands with palms up, denoting an openness to receive information.

All of these gestures matter in the exchange between patient and doctor.

Cultural differences may dictate some gestures and postures. One culture might show expressiveness, while another one might show constraint. Speaking tone and volume, as well as facial expressions, vary from culture to culture (Diversity Council, 2008). For example, people in some cultures use minimal expression, while others tend to express grief, sadness, or disappointment in a more open, demonstrative manner. Both the patient and the doctor should remember to be aware of these differences and be attuned to them.

"A physician is obligated to consider more than a diseased organ, more even than the whole man – he must view the man in his world."

— Harvey Cushing

What's Culture Got To Do With It?

Everything! A patient presents to a hospital, emergency room, or a doctor's office with a specific medical complaint. That patient brings certain lifestyle behaviors, cultural mores, and practices with him or her. Also, the patient has certain beliefs and customs regarding health and well-being, as well as thoughts and values about how health and disease are viewed. Needless to say, a patient's ideas and opinions about health and disease are influenced by numerous cultural factors, many of which are unspoken.

Culture determines human behavior. Our beliefs, values, and attitudes dictate how we respond to our specific circumstances and challenges. Our world is very diverse. Today, private practices and hospital systems serve more heterogeneous groups of patients than ever before. This diversity compels us to value different ethnic, religious, and cultural differences.

As physicians, we know that doctors and health care personnel have their own cultural and social biases, values, and beliefs about health, which they bring to the medical encounter. So, not only should the doctor value the patient's beliefs and cultural mores, but it should also work the other way around. Health care professionals must acknowledge and assess their own beliefs, values, and culture and not let these influence access to care, treatment recommendations, decision-making, or the willingness to consider alternative methods of treatment.

In the health care arena, it is critical that medical professionals recognize and address cultural and language differences in order to be effective in the delivery of medical services. Cultural sensitivity on the part of health care professionals is an essential component of patient-centered health care (Tucker, 2011). Health care systems and managed care organizations today require their medical staff and ancillary personnel to incorporate this sensitivity into their delivery of health care.

A study designed to look at patient-centered health care for the treatment of asthma found that patients who were treated by doctors or health care practitioners who spoke the patients' preferred language resulted in improved medication compliance, decreased emergency room visits, and a reduction in missed appointments (Morasch, 2005).

We believe that the emphasis on mastering cultural sensitivity will surely result in enhancing patient satisfaction, improving compliance, and fostering mutual respect between patients and health care professionals.

What Should Patients' Cultural Sensitivity Checklist Include?

As a patient, you must make certain that your health care professionals demonstrate:

o   Respect for all patients, regardless of religion, socioeconomic status, class, sexual orientation, age, or gender.

o   An understanding and acceptance of your rights as a patient to participate in medical decision-making affecting your health.

o   Acceptance of health beliefs and practices from other cultures that can be included into treatment plans, if feasible.

o   An awareness or acknowledgment of their own

personal beliefs that may interfere with their delivery of quality care.

There are a few signs that will give you some insight into whether or not your doctor values the concept and practice of cultural sensitivity:

o   Diversity in the medical office staff.

o   The availability of interpreter services.

o   Access to medical forms and educational materials in more than one language.

o   Medical interviews that include questions about your social and cultural practices.

It might be a big order to expect doctors and other health care professionals to comply with practices and behaviors to ensure cultural sensitivity. But the one thing we know is that when patients are in a trusting and non-judgmental environment, communication is likely to be at its best. Does this sound like the doctor has a lot to juggle in order to deliver quality patient-centered health care? You bet it does!

"Think like a wise man but communicate in the language of the people."

— William Butler Yeats

The Language of Medicine: Medical Jargon

Most professionals use a sort of verbal shorthand to communicate with their peers and other colleagues. This type of communication usually consists of abbreviations and acronyms that may be specific to the particular discipline. Medicine has its own jargon, which can present significant barriers to communication with patients (AMA, 2013). However, this jargon has a purpose: As doctors, we are trained to obtain factual information in order to determine or identify medical conditions, and then document and communicate this data to other health care professionals in a readily recognized manner. This is the *language of medicine.* It allows doctors and other medical practitioners to utilize a common language to understand a medical issue and facilitate collaboration across medical specialties. It may seem that doctors deliberately choose incomprehensible language to exclude patients, but in fact the sheer volume of medical information dictates that physicians take shortcuts by encoding verbal information. This can cause doctor-patient communication challenges. The need to provide clarity and decode medical jargon is an important factor in improving all health-related interactions. Why? Because clear communication and a confident understanding of a medical condition ensures patient adherence.

Some examples of medical jargon are the use of abbreviated terms, such as *ETOH* (which means "alcohol"), *p.r.n.* ("as needed"), and *b.i.d.* ("twice a day"). Doctors also use medical terminology such as *cellulitis* for inflammation of the skin, *dyspnea* for shortness of breath, and *dysuria* for painful urination. While these are common terms for health care personnel, this is obviously not the language used by the general public. These terms are not only universally recognized by health care professionals, but they actually describe the specific abnormalities, instructions, and/or observations of deviations from normal. In addition, these terms also provide shortcut directions for medication dosing. Despite the economy and utility of using jargon, it should not overshadow effective communication or patient safety.

Medical jargon can be unnerving, especially to individuals who do not speak English or speak it well. In any case, you should insist that your doctor translate medical jargon at all times. This will allow you to actively participate in medical decision-making.

The illustrations below depict a few of the commonly used medical abbreviations and acronyms.

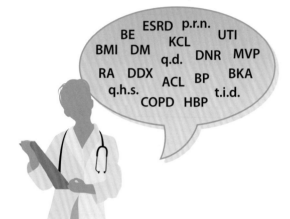

Illustration 1: Abbreviations used verbally and written. (See Glossary for interpretations.)

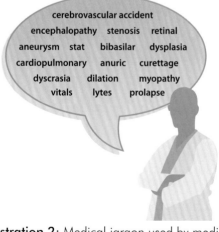

Illustration 2: Medical jargon used by medical professionals. (See Glossary for definitions.)

Medical terminology is becoming more familiar to the mainstream audience because of the plethora of medical and forensic television shows. Nevertheless, we cannot assume that all health care consumers have a working knowledge or clear understanding of that jargon. Take a look at how one doctor reported a patient's medical condition to a family member:

> "Your mother's recently diagnosed *End Stage Renal Disease* secondary to poorly controlled hypertension and diabetes now makes her a candidate for *hemodialysis*. Her *BKA* will make it difficult for her to get to and from the dialysis unit, so we will refer you to patient transportation services."

This is not only an example of poor communication with excessive use of medical acronyms and jargon, but there is no attempt on the part of the doctor to define medical terminology or explain cause and effect. While this was not done intentionally to confuse the patient or family members, this is the way doctors communicate with each other. However, if you don't interrupt doctors and ask them to break down the jargon and speak in lay terms, you will walk away without a clear understanding of the diagnosis or the treatment plan. So how can informed decision-making take place in the face of excessive medical jargon?

Here is a suggested alternative way to communicate the previous information:

"I would like to review with you your mother's medical conditions to make sure you understand her needs for medications and other treatments. She has poorly controlled diabetes and high blood pressure, both of which have caused her kidneys to fail. The kidneys filter toxins out of the blood and make urine. When the kidneys fail, this is called end stage renal or kidney disease, and is typically not reversible. It is a serious problem, but one that we are very familiar with, and it can be treated with a process called dialysis. This is a treatment performed 3 times a week for 3 to 4 hours at a special facility. The dialysis machine is like an artificial kidney. Because of the need for frequent visits and the fact that your mother has a below-the-knee amputation (BKA), we want to make you aware of transportation services that are available for her."

As you can see, this version takes a little more of the doctor's time, but this important message is communicated in language that the family is more likely to understand. It also paints a clear picture of the loss of function and what can be done to manage the disease. Eliminating the jargon will not only increase the family's understanding of the disease and treatment plan, but the family can also lend support to improve patient compliance. Indicating that this medical situation is a familiar one to the treating doctors can be very reassuring to the patient and family. In addition, informing the patient and family about transportation resources can be very helpful to them.

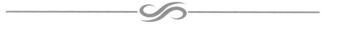

The practice of using acronyms and abbreviations in medical settings presents patient safety issues. That's why regulatory agencies such as JCAHO (Joint Commission on Accreditation of Healthcare Organizations) have set guidelines restricting the use of abbreviations that might result in adverse events for patients.

Imagine an order for a medication written by a doctor who instructs the nursing staff to administer a measured dropper of a liquid medication to an elderly patient "q.o.d." In medical language, this means "every other day," but it could be misread as "q.i.d.," which means "four times a day." Depending on the penmanship of the prescribing doctor and the knowledge and/or inquisitiveness of the administering nurse, the patient could receive the medication four times a day or every other day. Such confusion caused by the use of abbreviations could prove catastrophic or even fatal for some patients. Potential prescribing errors such as this, caused by illegible handwriting, should be eliminated by the use of electronic medical records.

In the nursing profession, there is a mantra called *the five rights: the right dose, right drug, right patient, right time,* and *right route.* Before administering medicine, an attentive nurse will be sure to have the correct information about these five factors.

As you can see, even among health care professionals the use of abbreviations and acronyms can be fraught with risks. So, when patients are sent home or discharged from the hospital without decoded information and a clear understanding of how to take the medications prescribed or how to follow any other medical instructions, you can imagine the problems that might arise. Your responsibility as a patient is to insist that the meaning of the acronyms and abbreviations be decoded into plain English at all times. The responsibility is on the health care practitioner to decipher the *language of medicine* and share information with the patient in a way that is clear, concise, and understandable.

As a general guideline, doctors or medical practitioners should confirm that their patients understand the diagnosis, treatment options, and medication dosing by having them repeat the information and instructions in their own words. There are extenuating circumstances to each case, and the complexity of some medical conditions may require more in-depth and ongoing discussions as the treatment plan progresses. Patients should request a written description or fact sheet of their medical condition, details of the treatment plan, and instructions on dosage and the schedule for taking all medications.

New Prescription? Now What?

We strongly urge you to review both the treatment plan and medications, especially when managing a chronic condition. Consider the case of a highly compliant but busy executive who failed to get a clear understanding of what medications he should be taking...

From Our Case Files...

A 48-year-old investment banker, B.H., was being treated for high blood pressure with Lisinopril 10 mg and Toprol XL 50 mg in the morning, and metoprolol 25 mg at bedtime. The patient had been taking these three medications since his last visit to his doctor. Before that visit, he only took metoprolol 25 mg at bedtime and Lisinopril 10 mg in the morning. On these two medications, his home blood pressure monitoring was normal. But his doctor noted progressive elevation of his blood pressure in the office. This prompted the doctor to increase the medications to gain better control of B.H.'s blood pressure. A prescription was written for Toprol XL 50 mg to take once per day. The patient took the new prescription to the pharmacy and started his new medication, along with the two other medications that he had already been taking for blood pressure control. One evening while packing for a trip, he asked his wife to bring all his bottles of medicine into the room where he was packing his clothes. She, being a medical professional, looked at the bottles and discovered that he was now taking three medications. When she asked her husband if he had experienced any light-headedness, he denied it. Then she asked him if his blood pressure had been extremely high on his last visit to the doctor. To this he reported, "No, just slightly elevated." At that point, she took his blood pressure, which was lower than his usual recordings. On close questioning, she discovered that he was more fatigued than usual, and informed him that he might be taking too much medication. She wondered if the primary care doctor had asked him to stop the metoprolol when the Toprol XL had been started. B.H. insisted that he only took medications as prescribed, and that he was taking exactly what his doctor had asked him to take. Fortunately for B.H., he was scheduled to see the doctor the following day before he left town. At his appointment, when he asked the doctor about the metoprolol and the Toprol XL, the doctor responded that B.H. should not be taking both the Toprol XL and the metoprolol, and that he should stop the metoprolol immediately.

What is the lesson here? Mistakes are unavoidable. But we can mitigate them with knowledge and thoroughness. At each medical visit, we urge you to bring all prescribed and over-the-counter medications and supplements for your medical practitioner to review. And, as a teach-back, you should review all medications and their dosages before leaving each office visit, especially if there have been medication changes.

Do not leave your doctor's office without an undisputed understanding of what to take and how to take it. The importance of making time for teach-back cannot be overemphasized. Teach-back is done by repeating the instructions to your doctor concerning medication, dosage, and dosing times. B.H. was lucky that he paid attention to his symptoms and his blood pressure had not dropped enough to cause fainting, or a fatal occurrence. He was also fortunate to be in an environment where he had access to an "on-call doctor," his wife. When B.H. was urged to follow his doctor's intended prescription, he gradually regained his energy and was back to his normal baseline in a few days.

Nine out of 10 patients have trouble following medical advice because it is incomprehensible to them. The risk of medical errors increases when patients do not clearly understand instructions. Remember, there is no margin for error when it comes to your health.

Informed Consent

Effective communication is most critical when patients must give informed consent. This type of permission is required before patients undergo a procedure, begin a treatment program such as radiation or chemotherapy, or participate in a clinical trial. This requirement does not apply to all medical procedures or treatments, but there are a few that you should be aware of which require your approval and authorization with your signature.

A list of invasive procedures would include but not be limited to:

o   Biopsy of organs or tissues.

o   Injections/aspiration of joints, spine, or tissue.

o   Catheterizations for cardiac or lung conditions.

o   Imaging procedures such as MRI, CAT scan, and PET scan (see Glossary).

o   General or specialized surgical procedures of any kind.

A list of non-invasive or minimally invasive procedures would include but is not limited to:

o   Echocardiograms.

o   Ultrasound.

o   Exercise stress test.

o   Colonoscopy/Endoscopy.

o   Cystoscopy.

> ## *Your Checklist for Informed Consent*
>
> ❑ Diagnosis or medical condition.
> ❑ Need for the procedure or treatment.
> ❑ Risk, side effects, and complications.
> ❑ Benefits of the procedure or treatment and consequences if not done.
> ❑ Discussion of alternative options.

What About the Anesthesiologist?

In addition to being informed about your medical procedure or treatment, you should be aware that all invasive procedures require anesthesia. It is critical that your effective communication with your anesthesiologist be a part of your preparation for any procedure requiring these services.

We share the opinion with many others that the anesthesiologist clearly plays a critical role in your surgical experience. Surgeons are often applauded for a successful cardiac bypass or removal of an appendix. However, they could not perform their surgical procedures successfully without the expert skills and intensive engagement of anesthesiologists. From Caesarean section to vaginal delivery, to removal of an appendix, to knee surgery, the anesthesiologist is there from beginning to end.

Therefore, your understanding of the anesthesia involved in your procedure is essential. The information below should be communicated directly to you by the anesthesiologist, who will be in charge of that aspect of your care. Your informed consent will also be required for the anesthesia. Furthermore, you should understand:

o   What type of anesthesia is being recommended.

o   What the potential side effects are.

o   How you will feel following the anesthesia.

o   What assistance, if any, you will need following the procedure.

According to the American Medical Association (2013), informed consent means that you, the patient, have sufficient information to make a decision regarding your body and health care. Any communication about your informed consent should be between you and the doctor who will be performing the procedure or instituting the treatment. It is the ethical and legal responsibility of the doctor to make certain that you are well informed.

Technology: Expanding the Reach of Clinical Medicine

Doctors who entered medical practice in the early years

of the twentieth century never imagined that a telephone and a computer monitor could be a major resource and tool in the delivery of health care. Telemedicine, the use of electronic communication and technologies, is one of the earlier technologically enhanced ways of providing health care and sharing medical information and expertise.

The concept of telemedicine is a product of the mid-twentieth century. It was initially created to offer medical services to patients who lived in rural areas where specialty care was not easily available. Specialists could review x-rays or pictures of skin rashes or eye conditions, make a diagnosis, recommend treatment, or suggest further evaluation. This technology, formerly referred to as videoconferencing, offered patients and health care practitioners the opportunity to address key concerns with convenience, privacy, and real-time, face-to-face contact. As the technology has improved and use has expanded, it is now known as telehealth in many circles. The video aspect of telehealth has provided improved and increased access to care for many patients.

In addition to providing access to specialty care that may not be available in remote areas, telehealth also saves time for the patient and doctor. Neither party is required to travel long distances to achieve an in-person, face-to-face medical encounter, and the expense of travel can be minimized. While some patients still value appointments in a doctor's office, many patients are quite satisfied with face-to-face contacts that lack a hands-on physical exam. For most patients, it's about getting the best care and being seen by an experienced doctor. Several studies have documented increased patient satisfaction with telehealth over the past 15 years (ATA, 2012).

Imagine going to your primary care doctor with a rash that is not easily recognized. Within minutes, you find yourself talking face-to-face via video with a dermatologist who can ask you pertinent questions and then observe, diagnose, and treat the problem, all within a 15- to 20-minute appointment. This certainly provides efficient and customer-focused care when the option is to wait three to six months to see a dermatologist whose office is 50 miles away. Telehealth also provides authentic privacy when a patient needs to be seen for a sensitive service, such as HIV care or a mental health concern.

Virtual Patient-Doctor Communication: A Time Saver, A Cost Saver

We know how difficult it can be for some employees to schedule medical appointments during a workweek, and many doctors' offices do not have late afternoon or Saturday appointments. For years, employers have been concerned that lost time at work for personal matters, including health issues, affects employee productivity, which ultimately affects the company's bottom line. With technology originally used for telemedicine to reach patients in remote areas for consultation and treatment, employers are now able to offer their employees virtual doctor visits. The employer pays a nominal fee per employee per month for this service. Typically, there is a medical assistant at the work site to assist with the medical visit by taking the employee's vital signs and noting the chief complaint. The employee is then connected via a computer to a doctor for a virtual doctor visit.

What a win-win! This innovative means of accessing medical care decreases the employee's frustration from traveling to and from the doctor, and both the employee and the employer save money. It also decreases the wait time to be seen by the doctor. The employee benefits by having minor medical problems addressed before they become serious, and by having convenient access to medical care during the workday. The virtual doctor visit can bring peace of mind to employees to have their concerns addressed immediately and without the worry of missing work time. The employer sees costs savings and less loss of productivity because employees can be treated in an efficient and timely manner, preventing the need for expensive urgent care or an emergency room visit.

Technology and Patient-Doctor Communication

The ability of patients to get their lab results online is a form of electronic communication. This technology is seen by many health care professionals as a way to avoid delays in informing patients of their condition and, in turn, avoiding delays in treatment. Health care professionals also regard electronic communication as a way of getting patients involved in their medical care. But since lab tests are usually presented without interpretation or explanation, they can be confusing to patients. Typically, lab work is not available online without prior review by a doctor. It would be ideal if laboratory results could be accompanied by a brief commentary that includes the doctor's assessment and any new recommendations based on the results.

Today, there is an increasing use of emails and texting between doctors and patients. This has added another dimension to communication for everyone, but it can be a problem for Baby Boomers (born between 1946 and 1964), who are still expecting their doctor to pick up the phone and call them or recommend another face-to-face encounter to further discuss medical conditions, lab results, or treatments. So, doctors are really caught between the old ways of communicating with their patients and the realities of the technology age.

Imagine a doctor with a multigenerational practice and the expectations of the Baby Boomers and the younger generations of patients. The Millennials, or Gen Yers (born between 1977 and 1998), are more likely to adopt electronic medical communication. This generation prefers less face-to-face encounters, expects and demands instant results, and thrives on texting, tweeting, and other instant social media communication. To them it is like oxygen!

It was only a few years ago that doctors began to be challenged by patients who used the internet as their primary resource of health information. This put many doctors in the position of being a source of "second opinion." While health information sites on the internet can be useful, the information can be complicated, confusing, and in some cases not even applicable to the medical condition that prompted the search. We recommend that this massive source of health information be used wisely.

Got a Medical Problem? There's an App for That!

Let's flip the script and put doctors on the offense. Many doctors use apps just as much as their patients do. So, why not capitalize on the popularity of smartphones to support disease management? Smartphone technology is being developed to address the biggest and costliest health care challenges. Diabetes is one of the first diseases to be targeted by the techies. According to the Centers for Disease

Control (2012), the cost of treating diabetes is rising; the latest calculation, in 2007, was $174 billion a year. Using smartphone apps to reduce the cost of health care by managing diseases such as diabetes, hypertension, and heart disease is very appealing!

So how does this work?

The patient can input laboratory or clinical information via a smartphone to his or her doctor, and the doctor can then respond with recommendations for further evaluation or treatment. Suggestions to refine existing treatment can also be transmitted. This could revolutionize the management of chronic diseases that are financially burdensome to the health care system. Solutions designed to get control of these costs are needed and welcomed.

Health and Wellness Communication Beyond the Exam Room

Support groups are not new to medicine. Many of them have evolved because of a need for patients with specific diseases, especially complex ones, to share their concerns with others who are facing or have faced similar challenges. Many of these groups are supported or sponsored by medical subspecialty advocacy groups, such as the American Cancer

Society, the American Heart Association, and the American Diabetes Association. These organizations can direct patients and family members to local support groups.

This form of health care communication has taken a giant leap. The health care needs of consumers have captured the attention of techies in a big way. The overwhelming embrace of social media by multiple generations is unquestionable, so consumers are now increasingly sharing their health concerns with friends and family members through their social networking on such sites as Facebook and Twitter. Social networks and chat rooms link users to discussion forums where many patients find a great deal of solace from knowing that they are not alone, and that there are people who can actually relate to their particular medical challenges. These groups, like in-person support groups, are extremely helpful in directing patients to various health care and self-help resources, especially for rare diseases. Patients actually rely on this information when they are considering where to go for treatments, which treatments are best, and how they can access special programs or clinical trials for complex diseases. Armed with this information, patients must then communicate their knowledge and concerns to their doctor. In turn, the doctor must be willing to be open to communicating and exchanging viewpoints with the patient – if time permits!

It is our firm belief that neither the information from support groups nor any technologically advanced methods of communication should replace the valued relationship and partnership of patient and doctor. We know that medical knowledge is empowering and that health literacy is essential to navigating today's health care delivery system. We also know that increased patient knowledge will put more demand on doctors and other health care professionals, requiring them to communicate more effectively, listen more actively, be less judgmental, and, in general, be more engaged during medical encounters. That is a big order. Why? Because the shrinking capacity of doctors and health care professionals to devote time to accomplish this is already evident, and will get worse as the number of patients increases and the number of doctors decreases.

Seeking Self-Service Health Care? It's Here!

Self-service health care kiosks are yet another technological advancement whereby patients can get vital signs monitored, have cholesterol tested, and even become enrolled as potential bone marrow donors. These kiosks, which look like ATMs and are often conveniently located in malls or pharmacies, provide a form of technology-based communication. They are designed to reduce the time and cost of health screening or routine doctor visits.

Our traditional training as doctors is hands-on, with a critical emphasis on the physical exam, which we still consider highly important. Nevertheless, self-service kiosks provide an innovative way to utilize doctors as well as an avenue to increase patient access to health care.

From a health care delivery standpoint, this technology is most attractive when you consider the current shortage of primary care doctors and the increased demand when 40 million people become eligible for health care coverage under the Affordable Care Act (ACA, 2010).

The Distractions of Modern Medicine

There are more serious time constraints and responsibilities placed on doctors and other health care practitioners today than ever before. The average primary care doctor sees one patient at least every 15 minutes.

The expanded administrative and supervisory roles required of many doctors are contributing to gaps in communication with patients and with other health care professionals. One time-consuming responsibility for doctors today is supervising physician "extenders," such as medical assistants, physician assistants, nurse practitioners, and certified nurse midwives. This expanded use of allied medical personnel has increased patients' accessibility to care, but at the same time increased doctors' workload.

For example, a few years ago, medical assistants were typically assigned to work the front desk, check in patients, perform vital signs, and then transfer the patients to the treating doctors. Now, medical assistants are performing breathing treatments, administering injections, performing EKGs, and, in some settings, performing ultrasound examinations, all under the license of a doctor, presumably under the doctor's supervision. Physician assistants, nurse practitioners, and certified nurse midwives function with full schedules and patient loads, just as doctors do: they take histories, examine patients, order tests, make diagnoses, and prescribe medications.

The scope of practice and responsibilities of mid-level health care practitioners can vary from state to state. While these health care professionals are essentially functioning as doctors, many states require medical sign-off by a licensed physician. As a result, supervising doctors may be required to respond to questions and consult on medical cases throughout the day, while seeing their own patients. These added responsibilities have contributed to the distraction and divided attention of both doctors and their staffs. These distractions, coupled with the need to be productive and provide quality patient care, make for a highly challenging and sometimes untenable situation for doctors.

Why is this important to you as a patient? These distractions pose limitations on your doctor's time and attention, posing significant barriers to effective communication. Keep in mind that while these medical services are being performed by allied medical personnel, the quality and standard of care is the absolute responsibility of the doctor of record.

Own Your Health Care

The practice of medicine, at its best, requires clinical competency, attentiveness, precision, and the utmost accuracy in making a diagnosis, ordering appropriate testing, and prescribing medications. The added responsibilities and distractions that burden doctors will not be resolved any time soon, because of increasing patient loads, the challenges of treating chronic diseases, and inadequate reimbursement.

Therefore, it is your responsibility as a patient to be diligent, informed, and intentional about your personal health care.

Your ability to understand your medical condition, follow medical instructions, and make appropriate health care decisions can only be accomplished through communication that is accurate, clear, honest, non-judgmental, safe, and culturally sensitive. As a patient, you seek medical attention because of a concern about your health. Your doctor invests time and resources to see you. You may or may not be in pain, but your health is interfering with your normal pattern of living. You pay for health care insurance, and your expectations for resolving your medical issues satisfactorily should be high. Why not optimize these encounters by ensuring that you communicate the most accurate and concise information to your doctor in order to receive an accurate diagnosis and proper treatment in a timely manner?

What's Next in Doctor Communication Skills?

We know as physicians that a significant emphasis has been placed on doctor-patient rapport, as well as the value of skillfully eliciting pertinent medical information during history-taking. While medical training programs prior to the mid-twentieth century did not have formal courses in doctor-patient communication skills, medical students patterned their doctor-patient encounters by observing and modeling the "bedside manner" of their professors and mentors.

So what happened to cause a breakdown in effective doctor-patient communication and engagement?

Decreased reimbursements, increased patient volume, and restrictions on time spent with patients, as well as the necessity to document encounters electronically, have all added to the decline of genuine and meaningful doctor-patient communication.

As we have already shown in various ways, the issue of health-related communication is essential, yet so complex. The ways in which a doctor elicits information from a patient and relates information to a patient are critical. Studies show that doctor-patient communication at its best results in: (1) acknowledgment of the medical problem; (2) improved patient understanding of treatment options; (3) willingness on the part of the patient to modify behavior; and (4) improved compliance with medications and disease management (Stewart, 1995).

Medical school administrators worry that the crops of freshly minted physicians they send into the health care world each year are not equipped with the "people" skills needed to provide quality patient-centered health care. In addition, these administrators are concerned about the role that poor communication plays in deaths due to medical errors. This has prompted medical schools to make doctor-patient communication an essential part of the core curriculum.

One example of this is the New York University Macy Initiative on Health Communication (2002), a collaborative effort among NYU, the University of Massachusetts, and Case Western Reserve, whose goal was to develop a comprehensive health care communication curriculum. According to this study, 35% of medical schools were teaching communication skills in 1988, and 65% by 1993. Nevertheless, these skills still declined during the students' clinical years.

Some medical schools are taking significant steps today to address the issue of poor doctor-patient communication in preventable deaths. These schools include Virginia Tech Carilion School of Medicine, Stanford, the University of Cincinnati, the University of California at Los Angeles, as well as several medical schools in Canada. All of these schools have adopted a system of multiple mini-interviews (MMI), which was developed by Dr. Harold Reiter of McMaster University in Hamilton, Ontario. The intent of Reiter's system is to assess the communication and social skills of prospective medical school candidates. With these interviews, the previously named schools hope to find candidates who demonstrate traits that will result in a pleasant bedside manner and an attentive ear (Harris, 2011).

The ability of young physicians to develop good communication skills will require them to be active listeners and have the ability to work in teams. We look forward to the day when good communication and social skills are used on a daily basis to ensure patient trust, a safe environment, increased patient compliance, and improved clinical outcomes.

Medical Encounters of the Best Kind

Establishing rapport with patients includes fostering trust, empathy, and compassion. This is usually thought of as "good chemistry" between patient and doctor. In reality, medicine is truly an art as well as a science. Moreover, some philanthropists who agree with the benefits of a good bedside manner are directing their funding to programs that reinforce communication and social skills. For example, the University of Chicago Medical School recently received $42 million to improve practitioner's bedside manner (Johnson, 2011).

In the health care arena, effective communication is one of the most essential fundamental skills that doctors and health care professionals must learn. We challenge our readers to enhance your communication skills and to hold your doctor to the same standard. It is our hope that both patients and health care professionals make communication effectiveness a top priority. This realization, coupled with cutting edge medical knowledge and skills, should ultimately result in medical encounters of the best kind.

Communication Tips for Patients

1. Always fill out medical forms completely and accurately.

2. Take time to complete your patient information in detail, listing past medical history, family history, immunizations, allergies, surgeries, and emergency contacts.

3. Prepare your questions before your visit to the doctor.

4. If necessary, request a certified medical interpreter prior to your visit.

5. Politely request that all communication be done in plain English, avoiding the use of medical jargon.

6. Relate your medical history in a thorough and concise manner.

7. Bring all prescribed medications and over-the-counter preparations to your visit.

8. Give an honest and complete history of when medications were prescribed or begun and how you take them.

9. When new medications are prescribed, insist that all your medications be reviewed by your doctor to ensure that old medications are discontinued, if necessary, or that similar medications are not taken.

10. When given medications, instructions, and a treatment plan, do a teach-back by repeating the information to

the doctor to confirm that you understand.

11. Be sure that you are given time to express your concerns.

12. Pay attention to body language – yours and the doctor's.

13. Do not tolerate repeated interruptions during your visit; reschedule if more time is needed.

14. Listen carefully to the shared information, take notes if necessary, and ask questions (Ask Me 3™ questions).

15. Recognize that listening is different from hearing, and active listening is the cornerstone of effective communication.

16. Review your EMR (electronic medical record) summary after each visit and correct any errors regarding your history or diagnosis.

17. Be knowledgeable about your medical condition, know how your condition will be managed, and understand the expectations from treatment.

18. Always ask questions when diagnostic testing is being ordered: What is the test? Why is it being ordered? How will it change my medical management?

19. Keep a Personal Health Record and update it on a regular basis.

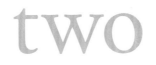

two

Navigating the Medical Maze

"The winds and waves are always on the side of the ablest navigators."

— Edward Gibbon

When we hear the word *navigation*, getting from point A to point B comes to mind. Charting a course from one place to another requires planning. In order to be successful at that, you need to know where you are and where you are headed. Navigation requires keen focus.

Nowhere is navigation as critical as in the health care setting. But navigating that system has many challenges – lack of a primary care doctor, timely specialty referrals, and insufficient medical knowledge, just to name a few. In general, inadequate understanding of how the medical care delivery system works and the challenges of medical insurance can cause significant barriers to you accessing medical care.

The Healthcare Landscape: Getting from Point A to Point B

Navigating the complex landscape of health care is hard enough when you are well. However, when you are ill and not at your best, you are apprehensive and anxious, which further complicates your ability to navigate health care issues. The uncertainty of the outcome conjures up feelings of vulnerability. You might wonder: How will this medical encounter impact my normal schedule, my family life commitments, my work responsibilities, and my life in general? This feeling of uncertainty can happen across the health care spectrum, whether you are going for an annual physical exam, a mammogram, or a colonoscopy. You can feel as if you are swimming in a sea of uncertainty, whether you are in a familiar or unfamiliar medical facility.

Add to the mix that some people find all medical environments highly impersonal. Stereotypes of formality, notions of not being included in the process, and dwindling trust in the medical profession have contributed to this sense of detachment. These factors can be barriers to establishing a healthy doctor-patient relationship. The recognition of the importance of patients' values and preferences regarding their health care is the basis of the new models of health care delivery that promise to be patient-centered. *Patient-centeredness* is the new mantra!

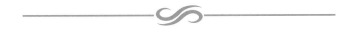

Let's take a look at one patient's experience. Sonia, age 42, went for a consultation with a breast surgeon for a newly discovered breast lump. "As I pulled into the five-story parking lot next to the office building," Sonia told her mother, "I wondered how I got to this point. Me, of all people – the health-conscious one – committed to an annual mammogram, and with no family history of breast cancer. When I got to the doctor's office, there I was by myself – all alone, with zillions of questions, as I waited for the surgeon to enter my exam room."

It's easy to understand why Sonia was stressed and lacked confidence at that moment. Navigating your way in an unfamiliar setting is often unavoidable in the quest to maintain your health or get the best treatment for what ails you. You may be anxious, apprehensive, fearful, cautious, and deliberate.

In order to successfully navigate most health care systems, you must be able to:

o   Select the right doctor for you and your family.

o   Know if, when, and how to seek appropriate urgent

care for you and your family.

o   Choose the best insurance plan for your health care needs.

Each of these areas can represent economic and access barriers to the best health care options.

The Right Doctor, the Right Reason, the Right Time

One of the most important decisions that you will make in your efforts to take charge of your health is selecting your doctor. We strongly recommend that the initial point of contact for patients be the primary care physician. That is the person you go to for your physical exams, preventive care, and referrals to subspecialists. We recommend that this medical professional be an internist, a family practice physician, or a pediatrician. Doctors who select these specialty areas are expected to master very broad and diverse areas of medicine. This allows them to recognize, treat, and manage a wide spectrum of medical conditions.

What happens when you require medical care, but you have not yet selected a primary care physician? Let's take a look at a case.

From Our Case Files...

H.M., a 45-year-old construction worker, out of work for a year, went to a dermatologist (skin specialist) because of a rash he had noticed for six months. Because he did not have insurance at the time, he ignored the problem. His first medical visit after getting insurance was to a dermatologist. Not only did he tell the doctor about the skin rash, but also about joint stiffness, knee pain, and stomach cramps. His exam revealed psoriasis (a scaly, patchy skin rash). The dermatologist noted that the patient felt pain when his joints were moved during the examination. Having no insurance, the patient had self-medicated with a number of over-the-counter drugs to relieve the pain, after which he began to have stomach discomfort. The dermatologist prescribed a treatment for the skin rash and strongly urged H.M. to see a primary care physician for his knee pain and stomach pain. The doctor further explained that the over-

the-counter medications, if continued, could cause a serious stomach problem.

What is the lesson here? Some patients fail to identify and utilize a primary care doctor as the first source of medical care prior to seeking specialty care. When this happens, we have seen many clients become frustrated in their attempts to be diligent about their health care. While H.M.'s decision to seek medical care for his rash from a dermatologist was reasonable, it is likely that a first-time visit to a primary care doctor would have resulted in not only a diagnosis of his skin rash, but also his other conditions. This is what a primary care doctor is trained to do.

How Do You Get Started?

A major source of physician referral has been and continues to be "word of mouth." Patients who have experienced medical care firsthand and are familiar with the bedside manner of a doctor are the best promoters or critics of that health care practitioner. A survey of 17 million adults in 2007 found that fifty percent of individuals in the United States selected a new primary care doctor based solely on recommendations from friends and family members (Tu, Lauer 2008). We know that many patients use a variety of sources, but the internet has become extremely popular for physician referral seekers, especially among the younger generations. Doctor report cards are available online from a number of agencies, as well as reviews and critiques by individuals. We must caution you, however, that relying on anonymous reviews without any kind of accountability can invite abuse, usually from disgruntled people.

Our advice is to use caution when you rely solely on consumer critiques to select your doctor. However, the internet can provide valuable information about a doctor's training, areas of expertise, credentials, and professional and hospital affiliations.

Why Is It So Difficult to Find a Primary Care Doctor?

As we have stated before, primary care doctors include family practice physicians, internists, and pediatricians. In some instances, obstetricians and gynecologists serve as primary care doctors. The Association of American Medical Colleges (AAMC) projects a shortage of approximately 63,000 doctors by 2015, a number that is expected to more than double by 2025 (California Healthline, 2012). Since the primary care doctor is, in most cases, the first point of entry into the health care delivery system, this shortage will present a significant barrier to access for many patients.

Why the Shortage of Doctors?

The common reasons for the shortage of primary care doctors include the enormous debt incurred from four years of medical school expenses and the required minimum of three years of post-graduate training – two major factors that delay earning capability. Fortunately, some philanthropists are taking note of this tremendous financial burden and its effect on the supply of well-trained doctors, especially in primary care medicine. For example, film and theatrical producer David Geffen established the David Geffen Medical Scholarship Fund, which allows medical students at UCLA to pursue their choice of medical specialty training debt-free.

Aside from debt, other factors that contribute to the doctor shortage include high malpractice insurance premiums, low insurance reimbursement, the loss of autonomy, and long work hours, making work-life balance unattainable for many. While the majority of doctors choose their specialty based on their passion and interest, many select the more lucrative specialties.

Because primary care doctors are the lowest paid of all medical specialists, fewer and fewer medical students are choosing to become primary care physicians. In addition, our population is living longer, so the demand for well-trained primary care doctors will continue to increase.

Many primary care doctors are already seeing the effects of this shortage, given the limited time and attention they can devote to their patients. Volume and patient flow have not only become the drivers to sustain a viable private medical practice, but are also used to gauge performance in salaried positions. Primary care doctors typically work twice as long as subspecialists do, while receiving half the pay. It is easy to see how this translates into "burn-out."

What Does Burn-Out Look Like and Why Should You Care?

Burn-out is manifested by extreme emotional exhaustion, sleep deprivation, depression, moodiness, and low productivity (Shanafelt, et al., 2012). If we look at these symptoms in doctors, factor in the long work hours, financial stress, and lack of professional fulfillment, we see a perfect storm for lack of empathy, poor communication, and possibly diminished diagnostic and clinical decision-making. Any one or all of these factors can have a negative impact on patient-doctor relationships and overall medical management. *That* is why you should care.

Primary care doctors in the United States have a higher rate of burn-out (37.9%) than other working adults (27.8%). Furthermore, front-line doctors, such as general internists, family practice physicians, and emergency room doctors, have higher rates of burnout than dermatologists, pathologists, preventive medicine specialists, and pediatricians.

Out-of-Network, In-Network: Why It Matters

Check to see if the doctor of your choice is on your insurance plan's panel of physicians. This is more important with managed care plans such as health maintenance organizations (HMOs) and physician preferred organizations (PPOs) than with traditional health insurance plans, in which patients have more flexibility in choosing their doctors.

A physician who specializes in internal medicine, family practice, or pediatrics is ideally suited to be the primary care doctor to guide you through your health care journey. Seeing a doctor who is considered "in-network" – part of a panel of preferred physicians – can be a cost savings to you, since the billed charges will be covered by the premiums you pay. Managed care plans have been around for a while, so health care consumers in the regions where this type of insurance is prevalent are already familiar with the requirements, especially with the need for prior authorization for certain medical services. Keep in mind that there are nuances to these health plans, so make certain that you are aware of any restrictions that might affect your access to care when you need it.

Let's take a look at what can happen when you change your health benefit plan without paying much attention to the coverage details and guidelines.

From Our Case Files...

When A.G. saw her primary care doctor for an earache, she was given an antibiotic. However, after five days, there was no improvement. She decided to make an appointment to see her Ear, Nose, and Throat (ENT) specialist. But when she arrived at the office, the staff discovered that A.G. had changed health insurance plans from a PPO to an HMO, which had stricter guidelines regarding specialty referral. In order for the visit to be paid for by her HMO, a referral from her primary care doctor was absolutely required. Without prior authorization for this visit, the ENT doctor would not be paid. A.G. had taken a day off from work, and the doctor had allocated time for her to be seen, so it was a lose-lose situation for everyone. To make matters worse, her ear pain persisted. After A.G. followed the guidelines and procedures of her HMO, she was able, several days later, to see her ENT specialist with a proper authorization from her primary care doctor.

What is the lesson here? If you change medical plans, be aware of any restrictions of your new plan before you need care. If you intend to maintain relationships with specialists, make sure that they are on the preferred physician panel of your new health plan. Read the fine print. Getting prior authorization may require you to physically bring the documentation to the specialist. However, some HMOs will allow authorization by phone. This still requires more staff time to secure proper documentation before your medical condition can be addressed, thereby delaying access to needed medical care. A.G. might have avoided this bureaucratic nightmare if she had gone back to her primary care physician when the antibiotic didn't work.

Want More Access?

Private practice doctors and their staffs have been besieged for years by complaints from patients, who are upset because they have trouble getting timely appointments, have to sit in the waiting room forever, get rushed through the doctor's examination, and cannot reach the doctor after hours. As reimbursement for doctor services has decreased, patient volume has had to increase to meet the basic financial obligations of running a medical practice. This has required doctors to reallocate their staff resources, their face-to-face patient time, and their attention to the business of their practices.

One option that some doctors have offered to resolve access issues is a new practice model known as concierge medicine, which began to surface in the late 1990s. Also called VIP medicine, direct care medicine, and boutique medicine, this new model provides timely appointments, decreased wait times, and increased time with the doctor. The model is highly appealing, allowing doctors to practice medicine free from time constraints with a smaller volume of patients, thereby fostering more meaningful doctor-patient relationships. Whatever name this model goes by, it offers health care consumers more personalized care.

You might ask, "Is this personalized care affordable?" Our research shows that the yearly fee for this service can range from $200 to $5,000, depending on the services that have to be tailored to your specific needs. Some doctors have elected to devote 100 percent of their time to this type of personalized care practice. Others maintain a more traditional practice model, while offering this service to a limited number of their patients.

Is Concierge Medicine for You?

Who wouldn't welcome more personalized medical care that would improve access, decrease wait times, and allow longer visits with their doctor? Sadly, our current health care delivery system is not conducive to this type of medical care delivery.

Enrolling in a concierge medical practice does not mean that you do not need health insurance. Concierge medicine offers a personalized approach to your health care in out-patient settings. Health insurance coverage will still be necessary for hospitalizations, emergency room services, lab and diagnostic studies, as well as office visits, depending upon the retainer paid by the patient. Private primary care doctors who have embraced this new practice model have organized themselves into a national association called the American Academy of Private Physicians. The slogan for this organization is "Liberating the Doctor-Patient Relationship" (AAPP, 2000).

If you think that more personalized medical care is something that you could benefit from, we suggest that you explore this new practice model. Our main concern is that whatever health care delivery model you choose, it should be one that meets your needs and allows you to be fully engaged in your health care decision-making.

Vetting Your Doctor

There are a number of factors that should be considered when deciding what doctor is best for you. It is important to inquire if your doctor has attained board certification—that is, has mastery at the highest level of knowledge and skills in his or her area. However, this level of credentialing does not guarantee improved clinical outcomes or competency in areas such as effective doctor-patient communication or comforting bedside manners.

Doctor availability and office procedures should also be looked at when choosing a health care professional. In many doctors' offices, physician assistants, nurse practitioners, and certified nurse midwives function as independent providers of medical care. Because of the variable skill sets of these practitioners, you should be knowledgeable about the roles and services they may provide in your doctor's office. That may prove invaluable to you as you navigate the health care landscape.

It is important to know how the office accommodates patients with acute or urgent needs. To decide whether or not a doctor's office will be a fit for you, you should ask these basic questions:

o   If patients call during office hours with an acute problem, will they be referred to an emergency room or are same-day appointments available?

o   Are appointments ever available after 5:00 P.M. or on Saturdays?

o   In the case of emergencies, can the physician be reached via a phone service?

o   Is the doctor's medical practice covered by other doctors after hours?

o   How does the doctor work with physician assistants and/or nurse practitioners, if at all?

When you are well, none of this may be important. But when you are faced with an undiagnosed problem or pain, these service options become critical.

Need a Second Opinion?

Making choices about your health care and the care of your loved ones is a serious and weighty responsibility. It is your right to question any medical opinion or recommendation regarding your condition. It is also your right to be adequately informed about treatment options. There are numerous reasons why you may seek a second opinion. These include: (1) overcoming uncertainty about your diagnosis; (2) dispelling confusion about your treatment options, including surgery; and (3) reviewing biopsy or laboratory results. In order to be empowered to take control of your health, you must be informed. So, ask questions and request a second or third opinion, if necessary. It's your right!

When it comes to making decisions about your health, doctors must be guided by the scientific and medical implications of your condition. Other factors that might contribute to your doctor's analysis of your condition are the doctor's experience treating the medical condition and the resources available to him or her, including advanced testing and procedures and access to subspecialists.

In all cases, this decision-making process by your doctor may not resolve your concerns or allay your anxiety about your medical condition. A second opinion may result in a different diagnosis or treatment recommendation, or you may receive the same message, delivered with more sensitivity and compassion.

How Do You Tell Your Doctor You Want a Second Opinion?

Another bump in the road when navigating the health care system is knowing if and when a second opinion is appropriate and how to get one. Most doctors are not annoyed when patients ask for second opinions; they may even encourage it. Nevertheless, you should give your reasons for requesting a second opinion based on your knowledge, medical history, family history, or just simply your need for reassurance. This second opinion may help you feel more confident about your health care decision-making.

The second opinion may be as simple as being referred to a subspecialist or to a center of excellence. It also could involve your doctor asking for a second opinion regarding a biopsy. We have found in our practice that the reasons patients ask for second opinions are:

o   The diagnosis is a rare condition.

o   Their symptoms are not consistent with biopsy interpretation.

o The original pathology report may be inconclusive.

o There is no family history of cancer or hereditary diseases.

o They do not feel comfortable with the diagnosis.

The latter reason is reason enough.

Let's take a look at a case where a second opinion was requested. The patient belonged to an HMO, but insisted on an out-of-network consultation.

From Our Case Files...

I.P., a 61- year-old teacher, booked an appointment to see his new primary care doctor after changing health care plans. He had experienced a twelve- pound weight loss over the previous four months, which he attributed to eating more vegetarian meals, increased work load, and stress. Upon examination by the doctor, a small, non-tender lymph node was found in his neck under the chin area. I.P. reported that he had been aware of a lump in his neck for over 40 years and insisted he had not noticed any increase in the size of the lump. He had no history of recurrent sore throats, tonsillitis, mouth or gum sores. I.P. had always been a non-smoker. Because of the lymph node and weight loss his doctor referred him to the oncology (cancer specialty) clinic. Following a review of his history and an examination, a needle biopsy of the lymph node was performed; the results were inconclusive. Therefore, an excisional biopsy (complete removal of the lymph node) was recommended. Analysis of the lymph node confirmed cancer. The patient was told that this cancer may have come from a salivary gland tumor. A total body scan performed, looking for spread of the cancer, was negative. The cancer specialist recommended radiation therapy.

I.P. decided to seek help from a surgeon friend because he was concerned about the diagnosis as well as the way the information was shared with him. His friend suggested that I.P. seek a second opinion. The second opinion doctor, who specialized in head and neck cancers, reviewed the patient's history, biopsy results, and total body scan report. The doctor was careful to explain the type of cancer, the recommended treatment, as well as the expected outcome. Unlike the previous medical encounter, I.P. felt more comfortable at this visit, because he was able to share his fear and anxiety about the diagnosis. While the patient was fearful of embarking on radiation therapy, he accepted the recommendation from his second opinion based on the doctor's approach, his detailed analysis and explanation of the benefits of treatment. Because the second- opinion doctor was referred by a trusted friend, I.P. was reassured and willing to proceed with the suggested treatment.

What is the lesson here? Always feel free to exercise your right to seek a second opinion especially if you feel that the diagnosis is not consistent with your symptoms. I. P.'s weight loss was certainly suggestive of a possible problem, but I.P. explained it away and attributed it to his life challenges and dietary changes. Fortunately, he did not hesitate to mention the weight loss, and it was a critical part of his illness history. A diagnosis of cancer is, for anyone, startling and frightening, and it is always best to get a second opinion if you are not comfortable. When faced with a new and potentially life-threatening disease, it is not unusual for patients to be concerned, confused and, perhaps, in denial. In many cases when the word cancer is mentioned, both the patient and family members go into mental lockdown. I.P. was fortunate that he had a trusted friend who could coach him and help him to navigate the situation.

So, Who Pays for Second Opinions?

It depends on the circumstance. In many instances, insurance companies will pay some percentage of the cost of a second opinion. Remember, a second opinion may require additional testing, that can be expensive and time consuming. Medicare will pay eighty per cent of the cost of a second opinion. If you belong to a Medicare HMO, it is considered your right to get a second opinion, but you will typically need a referral from your primary care doctor, and you must scc an in-nctwork doctor.

Tips for Seeking A Second Opinion

o   Request a second opinion in a timely manner to avoid delays in diagnosis and treatment.

o   Always check with your insurance company whenever a new treatment or consultation of any kind is needed, and especially if a second opinion is needed.

o   Inquire specifically about your financial responsibility for in-network as well as out-of-network medical care.

o   Always request and have in your possession your laboratory tests results, x-rays, scans, and any biopsy results.

o   Provide the specialist or second opinion doctor with your primary care doctor's contact information to facilitate communication.

Once you have decided that a second opinion is needed, following these recommendations should help you navigate any potential barriers that might arise.

You're Fired!

The most common complaint we hear from patients who fire their doctors is that the doctor does not listen. Failed communication is not only unacceptable, but it interferes with building a trusting patient-doctor relationship. This applies to both primary care doctors and specialists. Here are a few examples of inappropriate behavior that might alert you to a potential problem with your doctor:

o Lack of sensitivity or empathy.

o Rude or condescending attitude.

o Arrogance.

You should, however, be aware of more subtle signs that might affect your medical experience; warning signs that let you know your doctor might not be the right fit for you could include:

o Failure to respect your time (rescheduling, long waits, interruptions during the 15-minute visit).

o Use of medical jargon.

o   Lack of availability.

o   Consistently rude and unprofessional office staff.

In summary, the relationship between the primary care doctor and the patient is a unique one. There must be a sense of trust, honesty, and personal engagement between the two of you. The time, energy, and effort that you expend in the selection of your primary care doctor will pay off significantly in the long run. Your primary care doctor is the person with whom you should feel comfortable sharing your most intimate health concerns. Whether or not it is a good fit can be determined after a few encounters with the doctor, but may be sparked when you see the doctor in the office, face-to-face, on the first visit. Only then can you get a good feel for the dynamics between the two of you.

Firing Can Go Both Ways: Your Doctor Can Fire You

Yes, you can be fired. The usual reasons for doctors firing patients are:

o   Disrespectful and rude behavior on the part of the patient – it goes both ways.

o   Repeated no-shows and last minute cancellation of appointments.

o   Failure to follow treatment plans.

o   Non-compliance with medications, testing, and procedures.

A failed patient-doctor relationship can result in your doctor terminating your medical care. If this happens to you, it can be very unnerving and sometimes alarming. Doctors usually send a letter informing you that medical services will terminate after 30 days. If you find yourself faced with this situation, we suggest that you take action as soon as possible to seek a new doctor so that your medical care will not be interrupted.

Request copies of your medical records and be prepared to sign release forms for your records to be sent to your new primary care doctor. Resources that might be helpful in your search for a new medical doctor include the local medical society and specialty medical organizations. Taking these steps will provide you with the necessary emotional support you need and will facilitate your selection of a new doctor.

Please note that you can't be fired by your doctor based on age, sexual orientation, race, or religion – this is discrimination. We should mention a few instances in which it is not prudent for a doctor to dismiss you. These include, but are not limited to: (1) abrupt dismissals during ongoing chemotherapy; (2) a near-term pregnancy; or (3) some psychotherapy situations, where dismissal could adversely affect the patient.

In The Hospital...

While most of your contact with medical doctors will be in the out-patient setting, there will be instances when you may require in-patient hospital care. In today's health care delivery system, most hospital care is delivered by hospital-based doctors. These specialists are called hospitalists, a term coined by Robert Wachter, M.D. and Lee Goldman, M.D. of the University of California, San Francisco. This specialty description was originally published in the New England Journal of Medicine in August, 1996.

What is A Hospitalist and What Do They Do?

A hospitalist is a medical doctor, usually trained in internal medicine or pediatrics, who cares for you while you are in the hospital. These specialty physicians practice what is known as *hospital medicine*, and it is one of the most rapidly growing specialties in the medical arena. Hospitalists are available at the hospital to handle admissions, acute care, and the timely discharge of patients.

Most hospitalists are paid by hospitals or hospital systems, and the percentage of internal medicine physicians practicing as hospitalists jumped from 5.9% to 19% between 1995 and 2006. This trend has continued and it was estimated that in 2010 there were over 30,000 hospitalists (HPPartners, 2011).

It is clear from these numbers that the demand for hospitalists by health care delivery systems and hospitals is increasing. The increasing focus on quality of care and the efficiency of medical care delivery contribute to this demand. Proponents of hospital medicine argue that physicians who constantly care for acutely ill patients develop skills that make them better equipped to identify problems, to create treatment plans, and to move patients through the system quickly, thereby saving money for the hospital and health plans (Baker, 2006).

It is our belief that the appeal of the hospitalists is multi-factorial and not solely based on efficiency of care and cost savings. To the hospitalist, this specialty offers scheduling predictability, designated time off, and reasonable compensation. As this specialty of hospital medicine has evolved, many office-based physicians have embraced this specialty area because it has allowed them to be more efficient and productive in their practices.

The relationship between a newly admitted patient and a hospitalist is a critical one, and hospitalized patients can often be very confused about why they aren't being treated by their own doctor. We think that this might be a generational matter and can be attributed to a patient's expectations based on previous hospitalizations. On the other hand, there are patients who readily accept this model of in-patient care as special. For these individuals, they understand that the hospitalist is there to meet their immediate needs, and to coordinate their treatment plan. In order to bridge medical care for each hospitalized patient, these specialists must make every effort to work collaboratively with the primary care doctor.

What You Can Do To Help If Admitted to the Hospital

o   Notify your primary care doctor of your admission.

o   Request all medical records as soon as possible so that history, physical and diagnostic information can be reviewed.

o   Request details and outcomes of recent labs and treatments to avoid repeat testing.

Your Personal Health Record (see Appendix I) can be extremely beneficial to hospitalists because it will reveal chronic medical problems and details of your medications. After being hospitalized, it is advisable for you or a family member to contact your doctor about your hospitalization as stated previously. The ongoing communication between your primary care doctor and your hospitalists is essential. This will ensure that care for your new or recurrent medical condition is followed up appropriately and all necessary medications are acknowledged and continued.

While the use of hospitalists may provide more efficient acute care, it is not a panacea. Upon discharge, patients and their families must assume more responsibility for follow-up and continuation of medical care. The dictated discharge summary done by the hospitalist may not be seen by the primary care doctor within the first few days of discharge. Therefore, the burden is on the patient and the family to:

o   Schedule a timely follow-up appointment with the primary care doctor.

o   Sign a release form to ensure that hospital records are sent to the primary care doctor.

o Review with the hospitalist all medications and dosing schedules of medications with teach-back at the time of discharge.

o Ask which pre-hospital medications should be continued.

If there is a failure to follow through on any of these recommendations at the time of discharge, it could result in a perfect storm, leading to re-hospitalizations, and, in some instances, serious complications.

Discharge Planning/Post-Acute Care

We cannot emphasize enough the increasing communication and navigation challenges faced by patients and their families upon discharge from an acute care facility. Some of these challenges are: (1) scheduling necessary follow-up appointments with primary care doctors and specialists; (2) understanding activity limitations; (3) accessing transportation resources; and (4) arranging for in-home care, if needed. We know that successful recovery after a medical or surgical intervention is very much dependent on after-care. Not only is it in the best interest and well-being of the patient and their family, but it is the very best safeguard in preventing re-hospitalizations.

It's important that you and your family be aware of any post-acute care options in case your medical condition prevents you from returning home immediately following discharge from the hospital. Post-acute care can include:

o Out-patient rehabilitation care.

o Long-term care facilities.

These services cost and may not be covered 100 per cent by insurers, private or government subsidies. Again, the populations in most need of these services are the elderly and those with chronic diseases such as hypertension, diabetes, kidney disease, lung disease, and arthritis. Discharge planning should take place early in the hospital stay and you or a family member must provide input during this planning process.

Whether you are discharged to home or to an extended care facility, continuation of care is of utmost importance and it can potentially decrease your need for hospital readmission.

So, if you are physically and mentally able to actively participate in your discharge planning process, what should you do?

Your Post-Hospital and Transitional Care Checklist

❏ Ask your physician if a post-acute care facility will be needed.

❏ Ask a friend or family member for a referral, if a post-acute care facility is needed.

❏ Explore options for care in your community.

❏ Be knowledgeable about your diagnosis and treatment plan.

❏ Confirm that a discharge summary will be sent to your primary care physician.

❏ Ask what progress you should expect on a daily/weekly basis.

❏ Inquire about what problems might occur.

❏ Confirm which doctor you should call if a problem arises.

❏ Update *Your Personal Health Record.*

These recommendations need to be tailored to you or your loved one, and all follow-up measures may not be required depending on the complexity of your medical condition.

Let's take a look at a case that illustrates how important it is for patients to know what medications they should take and what dosing schedule they should follow when they are discharged from the hospital. This becomes even more critical when new medications are added.

From Our Case Files...

H.M., a 39-year-old male with a recent stroke, living with his mother, arrived at the doctor's office with his sister-in-law, reporting that he had no energy and sat around all day. He was being weaned off of prescribed medications for a mood disorder following his stroke. He had been discharged from the hospital two weeks prior with blood pressure and cholesterol lowering medications. On examination, he had a low blood pressure of 88/60 and when the doctor reviewed H.M.'s medicines, a bottle of his mother's blood pressure medicine was found. Neither H.M. nor his sister-in-law could confirm exactly what the patient was actually taking for blood pressure control. So, it is possible that the low blood pressure and lack of energy were due to his mistakenly taking his mother's blood pressure medications in addition to his own.

What is the lesson here? Patients who have had recent strokes or any disorder that might compromise memory, cause confusion or interfere with their *thinking process may require additional monitoring at home to guarantee that the treatment plan outlined at the time of discharge is being followed carefully. This unfortunate situation speaks to the fact that when patients are discharged from acute care facilities, they and their caregivers should completely comprehend all instructions regarding medications. This also supports the need for timely follow-up with your primary care doctor after hospitalization for review of your medications and clinical course.*

What could H.M. and his caregiver have done to help prevent his confusion?

Here are a few important questions that H.M. or his caregiver should have asked about his medications prior to leaving the hospital.

What I Should Know About My Medications

- o   What medications should I take every day?

- o   How often should I take them?

- o   How long will I have to take them?

- o   Why are the medications being prescribed?

- o   What results are expected from the medications?

- o   What side effects, if any, should I expect from these medications?

- o   Should I continue all of my old medications?

- o   Which medication(s) should I discontinue?

There are a number of ways that a patient or a caregiver can monitor medication dosing, such as accurately identifying each medication and assigning a designated day and time for administration of the pill. Popular daily dosing pill boxes are easily obtainable. This method of keeping track of dosing of medications can be used by anyone taking daily medications of any kind. Adherence to this practice will not only increase patient compliance but will help prevent medication errors.

Review of medications at the time of hospital discharge is an important part of post-acute care planning and your attention to the details of this planning process is essential to your well-being and your overall medical improvement.

Need Elective Surgery? Not in July

If you are hospitalized in July in a teaching hospital, there are a few things that you might want to be aware of. Teaching hospitals and academic medical centers provide state-of-the-art comprehensive care and high quality medical diagnoses and treatment. These centers are also the optimal settings for doctors-in-training to master their clinical skills and learn how to deliver the best care in the best possible way.

If you find yourself in need of hospitalization, whether for an acute problem or for an elective procedure, you will be subjected to protocols and a hierarchy of medical trainees and mentors – residents, fellows, attending physicians, and sometimes, department heads who may be involved in your medical care. We have witnessed the frustration of patients as parades of newly minted doctors, residents and fellows come to interview and examine them. This is an essential practice in teaching hospitals and academic medical centers, but it is crucial for patients to recognize some of the risks of being hospitalized in the month of July.

The repeated interviews and examinations by the new doctors-in-training can be a good thing. You will share your complaint(s) and your case will be discussed, reviewed and analyzed by more experienced physicians. This repetition of history telling, physical examinations, and case discussions should result in the best possible care for you. So, be patient with them.

But, there is a downside to all of this. The correlation between what has been called the July Effect (the influx of new interns, residents, fellows and the departure of experienced doctors), and an increase in medical errors, patient complications and deaths is controversial. Two studies by researchers at the University of California, San Diego and the University of California, San Francisco, have confirmed this association. However, a more recent study contradicts those findings.

The University of California, San Diego study

focused on fatal medication errors by examining 62 million death certificates recorded from 1979 to 2006. Of these, 244,388 deaths involved medication errors. The increase was considered to be a 10 per cent spike in errors occurring in July as opposed to other months and in counties with teaching hospitals versus counties without teaching hospitals (Phillips, 2010).

The occurrence of patient deaths due to medication errors is just one area that has been used to determine the impact of the July Effect. Mortality from procedures and efficiency of medical care delivery in the in-patient setting has also been examined. Researchers at the University of California, San Francisco, also looked at how the July changeover of doctors-in-training affects in-patient care. They presented findings from a review of thirty-nine studies, published between 1989 and July 2010, looking at mortality, efficiency, and quality of care. (Young, Ranja, Wachter, et al). These researchers concluded that, "Mortality increases and efficiency decreases in hospitals because of year-end changeovers." However, firm conclusions about the degree of risk, morbidity, and rates of medical errors could not be made based on the literature reviewed.

The Controversy Continues…

In 2011, researchers at the University of Tennessee Health Science Center in Memphis released an analysis of data on 12,525 surgery patients. The study found no difference in deaths or recovery times for patients treated in July versus other months (Krupa, 2010). It is clear to us that additional studies will be required in the future to support or dispel the validity of the July Effect.

What can be done to decrease medical errors in teaching hospitals in every month of the year? Our personal experiences as residents and attending physicians in community teaching hospitals and academic medical centers have led us to develop a few basic tips.

o   Try to avoid elective surgery during the summer months.

o   Know your medications and dosing schedules.

o   Be knowledgeable about your medical conditions.

o   If you can, try to distinguish the hierarchy – rank and file – of the medical team in order to target your concerns more effectively.

o   Do not be afraid to ask questions of any medical staff member.

o   Communicate, communicate, communicate!

Now that we have navigated some of the major speed bumps – choosing a doctor, the challenges of post- acute care planning and the pitfalls of hospitalization – let's explore the maze of scheduling appointments and getting to your destination to get the medical care you need. These may not pose significant barriers for all health care consumers but, for some, they can be monumental.

Another Maze to Navigate

A critical part of accessing medical care is scheduling regular appointments with your primary care doctor at times convenient to you and your family. If consideration of these conditions is not taken seriously, missed appointments or rescheduling can result in delayed and missed diagnoses, and ineffective treatment.

Let's consider the challenge of an employee juggling a work schedule and trying to book an appointment between 9am and 5pm. Work schedules present significant barriers to health care access. Many patients work long, protracted hours, and have limited lunchtime or breaks, making it difficult to see a doctor during a regular workday. Most doctors have limited early morning, late evening, or weekend appointments, thereby limiting options for employees. Because of this, employees will often forego routine health care visits. This potential barrier to needed medical care can be a challenge for all health care consumers, whether they are seeking preventive care or follow-up for chronic diseases. Failure to keep regular appointments can also lead to risky behavior on the part of patients who might engage in inappropriate self-medication and/or denial of symptoms. The tips below provide some viable solutions to these challenges.

Tips for Scheduling Medical Appointments

o   Have your health insurance card and any required prior authorization documents available before calling for an appointment.

o   Take advantage of online scheduling, if available.

o   Prepare a brief, concise description of your medical problem(s) that you can share with the scheduler (this may help you gain quicker access).

o   Know your availability and inform the office staff before attempting to schedule a visit.

o   Schedule early morning or very late afternoon appointments when possible.

o   Complete medical record release forms from other doctors prior to your appointment, when indicated.

o Be aware of your financial obligations for annual deductibles and co-pays.

o Inquire about interpreter services, if necessary.

o Confirm the doctor's or medical facility's address.

o Update *Your Personal Health Record* and bring it to your doctor's appointment.

o Keep and value regular visits with your primary care doctor and specialists.

Ticket to Ride

Because more medical procedures are being performed on an out-patient basis, hospital admissions have decreased and transportation needs have increased. This need puts an additional burden on patients and caregivers, who must take time from work to accompany patients, to insure the patients' safe return home. The lack of independence due to mobility challenges is, of course, greatest in our most vulnerable population – the elderly. Patients with disabilities and chronic diseases, as well as those who require multiple medical appointments, need dependable and timely transportation. Depending on the medical condition, public transportation may not be an option. For example, a patient experiencing urinary frequency would not be comfortable taking the bus or a van that makes frequent stops. A patient who has painful joints or muscle problems will have difficulty boarding a bus, therefore patients should solicit the help of family and friends, whenever possible, to assist them with transportation needs.

Solutions for Mobility Challenges

A valuable and trusted resource for patients and caregivers in some regions is the Easter Seals Transportation Group headquartered in Washington, D.C. This organization offers a free guidebook, *Transportation Solutions for Caregivers*, which includes practical tips to those caring for older adults (NCST, 2012).

Community Transportation Association of America is an excellent resource to identify medical transportation services. In some parts of the country, these services are known as "paratransit." Other transportation resources include:

o Faith-based organizations.

o State and community resources that provide day care services, taxi vouchers, and escort support.

o Government-funded volunteer driver services.

o Agency on Aging. (http://www.n4a.org)

o Eldercare Locator – a service that can give you a referral to local transportation resources for elders (www.eldercare.gov).

These are just a few resources that might be beneficial to you. We encourage you to explore other possibilities in your area.

Challenges of Navigating Medical Facilities

Have you ever gotten lost trying to find your way to a medical appointment?

Maneuvering from one department to another in a large medical center can be anxiety provoking. Some medical facilities with large parking structures will have a shuttle service to get you from your car to your doctor's office or laboratory and x-ray locations. Wheelchairs are usually available in most medical facilities and you or your family member should always inquire about transportation support in advance. While this may appear to be a trivial point, it is a potential barrier to accessing the care that you need when you need it.

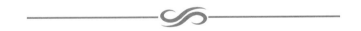

Headed to the Emergency Room?

One of the most challenging health care encounters you will experience is the emergency room (ER). This busy, fast-paced environment welcomes all-comers with various degrees of illness and can be very intimidating, whether it is your first visit or a repeat visit. People seek care in emergency rooms for a variety of medical issues, that may not be life threatening, because they are fearful and need reassurance. Patients go to emergency rooms for the treatment of colds as well as gunshot wounds, therefore it can be a short wait for some and a long wait for others.

The current economic environment – loss of jobs, loss of health insurance – has resulted in an increased use of emergency rooms for minor ailments, stress, and medication refills. These medical issues can be more efficiently addressed in your private doctor's office, a community health clinic, or a pharmacy. Other causes that result in the inappropriate use of emergency rooms can be job inflexibility, doctors' office schedules at capacity, and the failure of patients to keep regularly scheduled appointments with their primary care doctor. All of these factors impact access to timely medical care and they can, in some instances, contribute to a medical condition spiraling into an emergent situation.

According to recent government statistics, more than 300,000 patients are treated daily in emergency rooms in the United States. Before going to the emergency room, think twice about the urgency of your condition. Emergency rooms are designed to triage and see patients based on the severity of the illnesses/injuries. So, if you have a sore throat and other people are coming in with gunshot wounds, obviously, you will be seen after them. Do your best to assess the severity and urgency of your condition before heading to the emergency room.

Here are some symptoms that would warrant urgent attention:

o   Shortness of breath.

o   Sudden or severe pain.

o   Sudden difficulty speaking or walking.

o   Fainting, dizziness, or sudden weakness.

o   Changes in vision.

o   Uncontrolled bleeding.

o   Unusual abdominal pain.

o   Pain or pressure in the chest.

o   Disorientation, confusion, or changes in mental status.

o   Coughing or vomiting blood.

o   Suicidal feelings.

As we have previously emphasized, you play a role in how efficiently your medical condition will be addressed by being prepared. What can you do? Realistically, in an emergency situation, you may only be able to grab your medications. However, it would be helpful if you try to recall the onset and timeline of your symptoms in order to give an accurate medical history. Most importantly, whether your medical emergency is a recurrent problem or a new problem, a friend or family member should accompany you or meet you at the emergency room. Why? Because in a critical health crisis, you are compromised, and may not be able to recall your medical history, events leading up to your acute condition, or any other information that would help the emergency room team address your urgent need.

It is in the emergency room setting that an advocate can be most helpful. In this case, it can simply be serving as your support person or spokesperson. Typically, in a crowded emergency room, the squeaky wheel gets heard. So, your friend or family member can make sure your needs are addressed in a polite but assertive manner. There are a few crucial pieces of information that you or your advocate must know: (1) your medications; (2) your medical conditions; (3) your primary doctor's contact information; and (4) your insurance information.

Headed to the emergency room? Don't leave home without an advocate!

Is More Care Better Care?

Health care consumers are slowly beginning to realize that

more care is not necessarily better care. Acknowledgment of this can be a first step toward efficiently and effectively navigating the health care maze. As a first-world country, we are accustomed to demanding the "very best" and "lots of it," regardless of the goods or services. A person with controlled high blood pressure should not have to be cared for routinely by a cardiologist; nor should someone with controlled diabetes require regular care by an endocrinologist. Both of these medical conditions can be expertly diagnosed and treated by board certified internists. And yet, some individuals proudly boast about the treatment and care of their problems from specialists because their perception is that specialty care is "better."

Self-referral to specialists is a common practice; traditional health insurance plans and some PPO plans allow this flexibility for their enrollees. We are aware that when health care consumers over-utilize self-referral, fewer appointments are available for those patients with more difficult conditions who really could benefit from the services of a specialist. For example, the expertise of a cardiologist is more appropriately utilized in the treatment of complex cardiac diseases, rather than having a schedule filled with return visits by patients with controlled high blood pressure. The same holds true for other specialists like dermatologists and gastroenterologists, who can best use their skills treating complicated cases rather than having their schedules filled with basic medical disorders. While the desire to see specialists for a particular problem is tempting and preferred by many, we urge you to keep in mind that your medical issue can usually be managed by a well-qualified primary care doctor. This is what they are trained to do.

Pay Attention to the Procedures and Treatments Your Doctor Orders for You

A number of studies show that over the last three decades, doctors are ordering more and more unnecessary tests and procedures. This may be due in part to the availability of newer and better technology, but it can also be attributed to the fear of litigation. This fear has resulted in many doctors practicing "defensive medicine" to protect them and hospitals from lawsuits.

Almost everything we do in medicine has an upside and a downside. Doctors and patients must weigh the benefits versus the risks (potential for medical errors, side effects or untoward reactions). These errors run the gamut from allergies to medications, drug interactions, complications from minimally invasive or invasive procedures, and false positive results of studies that can lead to more medications, more procedures and even death.

It is for this reason that you must be aware of what tests are being ordered, why these tests are being ordered, and what potential complications could result from the testing.

Questions for the Doctor When Medications Are Prescribed

What does it do?

Why do I need it?

How will it help me?

How do I take it?

What are the side effects?

What side effects have you seen, personally?

How should I expect to feel while taking it?

How long must I take it?

What will happen if I stop taking it?

What will happen if I refuse to take it?

What are my options and what alternatives do I have?

Questions for the Doctor When a Test or Procedure is Ordered

What is the test?

What are you looking for?

Why do I need it?

How will it help my condition?

How will the results change your current decision about my treatment?

How must I prepare for it?

What are the possible side effects?

What are the possible complications?

What complications have you seen, personally?

How will it affect me afterwards?

What will happen if I refuse the test/procedure?

What are my options and what alternatives do I have?

Long checklists? Right. And they are worth every vowel and consonant.

"Medicine is a science of uncertainty and an art of probability."
— Sir William Osler

It's Complicated!

As the patient, you should be aware of the indications, the process, and the potential side effects of any testing or medical procedure. Having said that, we know that medical decision-making is complicated. We also know that medicine is an art and a science and that decisions are based on a combination of many factors. In today's health care arena, best practices revolve around evidence-based medicine, designed to manage disease based on proven protocols, methodology, and research. In addition, patient values and preferences are key components to incorporate into medical decision-making.

The final decision regarding testing and procedures ultimately rests with the doctor working in partnership with you. The doctor uses knowledge, experience, instincts, and expertise to make the very best decision that will produce the best clinical outcomes.

The Next Wave

As our health care landscape continues to evolve, no one knows exactly what accessing health care will look like in the future. As the limitations of managed care become clear, we are now witnessing the next wave of health delivery systems – Medical Homes and Accountable Care Organizations (ACOs). Federal dollars have been directed to medical facilities to set up the infrastructure for these new delivery models. These systems have a patient-centered focus and the push for active patient participation is coupled with sufficient patient education so that patients fully understand their disease, their treatment options, and the consequences of their decisions. These health care delivery models are designed to improve the coordination and quality of care, facilitate patient navigation, improve health outcomes and, ultimately, decrease medical spending. There are specific characteristics that these delivery systems must possess, regulations they must adhere to, and outcomes that must be fulfilled. The success of this new health care delivery will depend on proving the model.

What Has Happened to the Private Practice of Medicine?

The number of doctors entering the private practice

of medicine has diminished over the last decade. It is no secret that we are facing and will continue to face physician shortages. A few reasons for this are: (1) fewer people are choosing medicine as a career; (2) the financial burden of running a medical practice has increased dramatically; and (3) physician compensation continues to be stagnant. In addition, younger doctors are choosing to work fewer hours than their senior colleagues in order to ensure an acceptable work-life balance.

We have previously discussed in this chapter other causes of our ever-increasing doctor shortage such as overwhelming debt from medical school and post-graduate training, the uncertainty of the role of the doctor in health care delivery, and "burn-out." In order to comply with the required guidelines for reimbursement under most health care plans, doctors have had to expand their staff in order to fulfill duties such as: (1) securing prior authorization; for services; (2) documenting services and verification of coverage; and (3) transitioning to the use of electronic medical records.

Over the last twenty-five years, there has been a fundamental shift in how doctors manage their medical practices. In large part, this has been an absolute necessity for financial survival. In many parts of the country, doctors in private practice are not only responsible for managing their medical practices with all of the inherent liabilities, but they also face:

o The harsh economic reality of declining reimbursement for services provided.

o Decreased access to specialists.

o Increased responsibility of caring for the uninsured.

o Limited access to medications for patients due to health plan formulary restrictions.

Prior to the implementation of managed care, doctors in private practice operated largely as small business owners, taking care of their patients, and maintaining the trust of these patients through availability and the demonstration of personal concern for their patients' well-being. We know that there has always been a discrepancy between income for primary care doctors and subspecialty care doctors – gastroenterologists, surgeons, and cardiologists. However, delivery of care under the private practice model afforded most doctors a reasonable and comfortable lifestyle. There is no question that the added cost of doing business, especially for primary care doctors in private practice, has resulted in the adoption of more expedient ways of delivering medical care in order to survive financially. In addition, this cost of doing business will also affect your ability to navigate the system to access needed medical service which can ultimately impact the quality of your medical care. Therefore, it is essential that you partner with your primary care doctor, be intentional about your health care and value the importance of communication and navigation to achieve clinical outcomes of the best kind.

Navigation Tips

1. Know your health insurance plan and what services are covered for out-patient care and in-patient care.

2. When making your appointment, give a clear, concise main complaint so that a realistic time allowance for your appointment can be made.

3. If you know that your medical complaints/concerns will take longer than 15 minutes, plan to book a second appointment.

4. Journal your concerns over a few days before your doctor's appointment so that your history is accurate, concise and informative.

5. Know your medications and ask specific questions about dosing when new medications are added.

6. Ask your doctor to arrange for you to receive a copy of your lab results, if you desire.

7. Schedule x-ray and procedure appointments as soon after requested as possible.

8. Ask you primary care doctor about availability of same-day sick appointments.

9. If diagnostic testing (invasive or non-invasive) is recommended, be clear about your responsibility

for preparation as well as follow-through with these studies.

10. Ask about what you should expect regarding side effects, untoward reactions, or change in your activity.

11. If you are not clear about your diagnosis or have reservations about the recommended treatment, do not hesitate to ask for a second opinion or a specialty referral.

12. Try to avoid elective surgery in the month of July.

13. Always notify your primary care doctor when you are hospitalized.

14. Insist on immediate and ongoing communication with your primary care doctor and the hospitalist.

15. Understand your responsibilities for your care and know your medications, when discharged from the hospital, whether you are going home, to skilled nursing, or other transitional care facilities.

16. Avoid seeking care in an emergency room for a non-urgent problem.

17. Always, always have a family member or friend accompany you to or meet you at the emergency room.

three

Advocacy Appropriately Done

"It is not enough to be compassionate. You must act."

— Tenzin Gyatso

Now that we have shared with you the importance and value of effective communication and savvy navigation, we would like to focus this chapter on what we consider a critically important means of obtaining your best health through advocacy.

No other aspect of your life is more important than your health and well-being. Enjoying a state of wellness is essential for you to be a loving and supportive spouse, a giving and engaged parent, or a productive and visionary employee. We would now like to introduce a concept and practice that will enhance your health experience and, if done appropriately, contribute to the best medical encounters and clinical outcomes for you.

If the concept of advocacy seems familiar to you, it is. Children, elderly patients, and patients with chronic diseases are the most vulnerable consumers of health care. Parents advocate for their children on a daily basis – in the health care setting, at school, on the playground, and in social situations. They are involved in deciding what schools and teaching methods are best for their children. They go to parent-teacher conferences to share information and to receive insight into their children's progress. Children must be accompanied by a parent or legal guardian to doctors' appointments up to 16 years of age. While this is the law, it is a practical and necessary requirement, to ensure a meaningful medical experience. These adults serve as the spokespersons for their children. This is the type of patient advocacy that you most likely know about.

What Exactly Is Patient Advocacy?

Simply put, patient advocacy is assisting patients to improve their health care by assuring that they are well informed and that quality medical care is accessible to them in today's complex health care delivery system. Typically, health care consumers enter the medical system when their health is compromised. Under these circumstances, they are often least able to tell their medical story or deal with the challenges of navigating the out-patient setting, the hospital experience, or the emergency room. It is in such instances that a patient advocate can serve as the voice of patients when they are unable to think clearly, overwhelmed by the situation and not at their best.

The act of patient advocacy is not new, but this practice as a discipline is an emerging trend. The demand for such a service is increasing because patients face barriers to medical care and are challenged by complex insurance benefits and a variety of treatment options. Another reason for this demand is the increasing burdens facing doctors and other health care professionals, resulting in limited patient interaction time. Because there are so many medical treatment options today, about which patients have limited knowledge, more time is needed for doctors to explain and respond to patients' questions at a time when visits are becoming shorter and shorter. This situation is what drives many health care consumers to do their own investigations and due diligence, which in many cases can lead to more patient confusion.

Patient advocacy should not be reserved only for crises or acute medical needs. Health care consumers with well-controlled chronic conditions can also benefit from appropriate patient advocacy.

People are living longer these days, thanks to medical technology and health care advances. The subspecialty of geriatrics is dedicated to the treatment of the elderly. These subspecialists are proficient in addressing the special needs of the aging population. It is estimated that there are approximately 75 million baby boomers today, who are part of the so-called "sandwich" generation. According to the National Association for Insurance Commissioners (2012), these individuals are simultaneously preparing their kids to leave the nest, while caring for elderly parents and planning for their own retirement. Nearly 10 million boomers over the age of 50 are caring for an aging parent today.

We regard these sandwich generation boomers as patient advocates by default. They are continually seeking resources to lighten their burden of providing health care support for their parents – and sometimes their grandparents. Information, consultations, and assistance navigating the health care system are top priorities for these caregiving boomers. The demand for support in providing quality health care will become more prevalent as consumers are required to take on more responsibility for health care needs. Effective patient advocacy can bring clarity to the medical experience, improve compliance, and ultimately enhance clinical outcomes. But first, the need for advocacy must be recognized!

Why Patient Advocacy?

Why not? Adults consult with attorneys when they are confronted with a legal dilemma, real estate brokers for property issues, and financial advisors for estate planning and investment matters. Adults would never venture into these arenas without expert advice. In matters related to health, it would be ideal if we could depend exclusively on the recommendations and advice of our primary care doctors. That would be in a perfect world. However, there has been a sea change in health care delivery over the last twenty years, which has resulted in the need for health care consumers to be better informed and more assertive. When it comes to their health, people just think they can "go it alone." Therefore, they are insufficiently equipped to access appropriate medical care, understand their medical condition, or make informed decisions about what options are available to them. In most cases, this self-assured approach may work well for a number of years, especially if there are no urgent or critical medical issues. However, attempting to navigate the medical system alone when you are faced with multiple chronic conditions can certainly be frustrating, which is usually accompanied by insecurity and confusion. That is the time to consider the help of a patient advocate.

What Is The Role of a Patient Advocate?

A patient advocate is anyone who acts on behalf of a patient to help improve and maintain a high quality of health care for that individual. Patient advocates are important when illness threatens a person's well-being, independence, or ability to understand and engage in medical decision-making.

Patient advocacy at its best helps to alleviate fear and anxiety about the unknown, improves understanding of medical conditions and treatment, and paves the way toward good clinical outcomes. The patient advocate accomplishes these objectives by having adequate medical knowledge, demonstrating active listening, and ensuring that the patient understands his or her condition and responsibilities. We know of many instances in which successful patient advocacy has facilitated access to medical care, improved patient-doctor communication, prevented medical errors, and improved the overall medical experience. The following cases will demonstrate the value of patient advocacy in acute and non-acute medical settings.

The Burden of Multiple Chronic Diseases

High blood pressure, diabetes, heart disease, and kidney disease are the most common chronic diseases seen by primary care doctors. In many instances, at least two of these diseases occur in the same patient and must be addressed by the treating doctor on a continuing basis. The ability to adequately control these multiple conditions requires patient and family education, motivation, compliance, and access to medical care. The monitoring and treatment of individual diseases can be fairly straightforward; however, a combination of these diseases may require a balancing act by all the parties concerned. Depending on its severity, each condition may require simultaneous coordination of care by multiple specialists. Many of these patients are elderly and may not have family members with the time, desire, or interest to offer any assistance.

Approximately 66 percent of the American population had chronic medical conditions in the year 2000. Of that number, 21 percent had multiple chronic conditions. These numbers continue to grow as our population ages. In 2002, the leading worldwide chronic diseases were cancer, diabetes, cardiovascular disease, and chronic respiratory disease. Chronic diseases are major contributors to the escalating cost of health care. And yet, patients with these diseases are the most vulnerable. They are also the most at risk for medical errors. Why? The multiple medications they take, the difficulty of coordinating the various aspects of their care, and the challenge of their complying with appointments and testing can be overwhelming for anyone – regardless of their support system, health insurance coverage, educational level, or income. Patients find themselves caught in a web of uncertainty, lacking the knowledge of if, when, and how they should seek support or advice, and needing to depend on medical professionals who may be unfamiliar to them. This is prime time for patient advocacy. (Anderson & Horvath, 2004; Yach, Hawkes, Gould, & Hofman, 2004.)

Imagine a 72-year-old man with diabetes and end-stage kidney disease who receives his medical care at a large multispecialty clinic, where he has been assigned to a primary care doctor and a kidney specialist. He is also receiving kidney treatments (dialysis) at a separate facility. The patient lives alone in a two-story home and depends on his two adult children (when they are available) for food preparation, shopping, and transportation to and from the doctor. At other times, he uses paratransit services. The patient's most recent office visit showed a normal blood pressure, and blood tests revealed adequate control of his diabetes.

At first glance, it appears that this patient's medical care is under control, with stable vital signs recorded during his follow-up visits, compliance with dialysis treatments, and normal blood sugars reported on several recent visits. But let's take a closer look at some recent developments:

o   The patient was given pain medication at his last medical visit because of back and hip pain.

o The family noticed that he was sleeping more during the day.

o The patient complained of soreness of the skin on the back of his buttocks.

o The patient has recently required assistance to the bathroom.

Could this patient benefit from an advocate?

You bet he can! He seems to be on a slippery slope. An intervention by an advocate at several junctures over the last few weeks could have made all the difference in his sense of well-being.

Who could have been his advocate?

This patient could have benefited from advocacy by a peer, family member, home health aide, or professional patient advocate.

A peer advocate could have recognized this patient's increasing inability to get around and alerted the family or urged the patient to call his primary care doctor for advice. He could then have been encouraged to schedule an appointment because of the change in his ability to perform his usual daily activities. In this case, the difficulty was getting to the bathroom. Sometimes an advocate must take that extra step and, with the patient's permission, call to schedule an appointment for the patient.

When Compassion Is Not Enough, Act...

This case demonstrates how easily and quickly a patient's health can spiral out of control, especially when there are multiple medical conditions. A patient's understanding of his disease and its potential complications is key to better management, resulting in the best clinical outcomes. An assertive family member could alert health care providers to any new problems and insist on immediate attention. A trained patient advocate could have identified the problem, initiated basic care, and scheduled an appointment with the primary care doctor. However, given the unusual challenges faced by patients with multiple conditions – in this case, kidney failure, diabetes, hypertension, undiagnosed pain, limitation of motion, and bed sores – a professional patient advocate would have been in order.

Professional patient advocates (ideally, doctors, physician assistants, nurse practitioners, or certified patient advocates) have sufficient medical training to be knowledgeable about medical conditions and complications. They are also well versed on which medications are indicated, how they should be taken, and their possible side effects. With the patient's permission, they can work in conjunction with the family and the medical care providers to implement a workable plan for management of medical conditions and coordination of care. While most of this advocacy could be handled by a family member or a peer, cases of complex diseases might benefit from the support of a professional patient advocate. In all of these matters, professional advocates are expected to maintain all communications as privileged and confidential, to keep the patient well informed, and to always make patient safety the top priority.

Is Patient Advocacy for You?

It is always difficult to accept the reality of being limited physically or mentally, whether that is temporary or permanent, and whether the process is acute or gradual. The knowledge that your daily pattern of activities might change and that your lifestyle might be altered due to an illness can be extremely disturbing. You may be afraid, anxious, or in denial, which can interfere with your ability to relate an accurate medical history. In some cases, you may have little or no memory of the sequence of events that led to your decline in function. Can you recall ever asking a loved one or a friend who has recently had a medical encounter what the doctor said regarding the medical complaint? Did you get a response that assured you that your loved one or friend had a clear and informed idea of the diagnosis, indications for treatment, or options for management? Probably not.

Time and again, we have been told by clients that they have left a medical appointment without being able to tell their spouse or family members the outcome of that office visit. They often feel inadequate and unable to sort out not only the details of the encounter but, more importantly, what next steps they need to take in the management of their condition. In many instances, if patients present with a complicated medical condition, they are so overwhelmed by the idea of being physically compromised that they do not hear what is being said to them. Elderly patients are of particular concern because they typically have one or more medical conditions, for which they take a number of different medications. It is difficult for them to keep track of the various medications and dosing schedules. In addition, the added responsibility of getting the diagnostic studies required to confirm the working diagnosis can be daunting. These challenges are apparent in non-urgent situations; imagine what happens when there is an acute situation, and the patient is significantly compromised, perhaps because of severe pain, symptoms of heart disease, or symptoms of stroke.

As a result of our many years of advocating for our own children, relatives, and friends, we know that it is in the health care setting that patients fail to get a clear understanding of their condition, and that is when a trusted patient advocate can be invaluable. It is in this setting that patient advocacy becomes an essential tool to ensure that you and your loved ones can optimize your medical experience and attain your best health.

In some cases, a family member who is willing to be an advocate for a loved one can really make a difference. This person must be vigilant, compassionate, and willing to ask appropriate questions.

From Our Case Files...

H.S. is an 80-year-old retired electrician who experienced confusion following surgery at a local hospital. Prior to that, he had been in good health and engaged in a regular daily exercise routine. H.S. saw his doctor on a yearly basis and was not on any prescribed medications. He had been hospitalized once, 30 years before for surgery, at the same hospital to "remove a growth on his liver."

One month before his surgery, H.S. was admitted to the hospital from the emergency room, where he presented with four days of fever, weakness, and severe abdominal pain. A diagnosis of a ruptured diverticulum (an out-pouching of the colon) was made. He was treated with antibiotics, and a drain was placed in his abdomen for three weeks. A future surgical date was set for one month later.

One day after H.S.'s surgery, his wife found him to be incoherent, delusional, and mildly agitated. He *had been placed on narcotics via a patient-controlled analgesic pump (PCA) for post-surgical pain. When his wife reported his unusual behavior to the nurse and the staff doctor on call, she was told, "This is a normal reaction for someone his age." But she was not satisfied with that explanation, and insisted that H.S. was "not himself." Then she requested the name of the narcotic and went home to research it on the internet. She soon discovered that H.S. displayed many of the mental changes that were reported as possible side effects from this medication. The following morning, she called the surgeon and asked the staff for a review of all medications. When the wife questioned H.S., he recalled that he had experienced some confusion after his surgery 30 years before. At that time, his confusion was thought to be due to the narcotic used to control his pain. H.S.'s doctor then discontinued the PCA pump and made adjustments to his pain medication, after which H.S. experienced noticeable improvement in his mental state.*

What is the lesson here? Why was this patient's history of an untoward response to pain medication not easily elicited during his medical history intake? Keep in mind that H.S.'s previous experience occurred 30 years before. It is always helpful to have someone with you when you undergo a major medical intervention. A family member is most likely to be able to identify any unusual reactions or behavior, and can help you to relate your medical story. In H.S.'s case, it was advantageous that his advocate was his wife, who was not only able to get him to recall past experiences but also to research the side effects of the medication in question. She refused to accept the explanation given by the nurse and staff doctor, insisting that the root cause of H.S.'s confusion be found. This type of advocacy can be enormously helpful in today's in-patient hospital settings, especially in cases in which hospitalists are the treating doctors of record, and not the primary care doctor who is familiar with the patient.

We know you have heard friends say something like, "My mother was never the same after that surgery." It is well known that elderly individuals do not always fare well after a major surgery or invasive medical procedure. In many instances, simply a change of environment from home to a hospital setting can result in confusion, disorientation, and anxiety. Coupled with the effects of anesthesia and surgery, this can lead to an altered mental state, as was displayed by H.S.

Family members must be keenly aware that hospitalized patients are at risk for experiencing adverse reactions and post-surgical complications. Therefore, we recommend that family members should make every effort to be available to monitor their loved ones after surgery. This may go a long way to identify certain behaviors that might otherwise be dismissed by medical personnel as simply age-related.

Making the Case...

Health care consumers must be equipped with tools not only to *navigate* the health care system but to *communicate* their needs and desires to health care providers to ensure quality care and effective medical encounters. Sadly, in too many instances, consumers are not able to accomplish this on their own. That is when patient *advocacy* becomes essential.

Let's take a look at some startling statistics of patient-doctor encounters that we know could have had very different outcomes if patient advocacy had been an essential part of the medical experience:

o   Gogoi (2006) revealed that "50% of patients leave their physicians' offices not knowing what to do"; only 15% of patients receive answers to their questions during routine medical encounters; and 61% of the time patients choose the wrong type of specialist.

o   Jenks, Williams, and Coleman (2009) revealed that in 50.2% of the cases of patients who were re-hospitalized within 30 days of being discharged for any condition, there was no evidence that the patients had followed up with their physicians.

In each of these instances, appropriate patient advocacy could have served to alleviate or mitigate these unacceptable consequences. This will become clearer as we elaborate on the value and importance of patient advocacy.

We believe that patient advocacy at its best is always founded on the basis of giving patients the tools to ultimately advocate for themselves and their loved ones when they can. Again, the need for patient advocacy must first be recognized.

Let's take a look at how a busy urban professional caregiver was able to get a timely and appropriate referral for her mother with the help of a professional patient advocate.

From Our Case Files...

A.G., a practicing attorney who lives in a metropolitan area, has recently taken on the responsibility of caring for her aging mother, who has moved in with A.G. to be closer to her daughter. Shortly after that move, there was some urgency to get medical attention for the mother because she was becoming more dependent on her daughter for help with activities of daily living. Most of the mother's dependency was due to the onset of recent foot pain, which caused her difficulty in getting around.

A.G. was stressed by the added time commitment necessary to supervise her mother's condition. This additional time, combined with her inability to get an urgent appointment for her mother with the overbooked primary care doctor, led A.G. to contact a physician friend. The mother's foot pain began several weeks after a routine medical appointment with her primary care doctor, and had become more and more incapacitating. After talking with A.G. and determining that the mother's problem was limited to her foot pain, the physician friend recommended an alternative approach, advising A.G. to request a referral from the primary care doctor to a podiatrist (foot specialist). In addition, the friend suggested that the mother be evaluated for physical therapy and other ancillary services, such as in-home health support.

After the primary care doctor referred the mother to a Podiatrist, that specialist helped the mother to resolve her foot problem. As a result of A.G.'s discussion with her physician friend, who happened to be a professional patient advocate, A.G. was empowered and coached not only to insist on a referral but to take advantage of other medical resources.

What is the lesson here? This busy urban professional recognized that she needed help. As a result of this, she was coached by her physician friend on how to effectively communicate her needs to the doctor and staff and navigate the system to get the needed care for her mother. Not only was A.G. redirected to get the most appropriate care for the urgent foot problem in order to avoid further complications, but she was also educated about the need to pursue other home health resources that her mother was eligible for. The outcome of this engagement with a professional patient advocate gave A.G. the tools to significantly assist her mother. It also gave her the comfort and relief that she needed in order to resume her busy and demanding lifestyle and to be productive in her profession.

This case represents the value of professional patient advocacy. The acute problem was addressed in a timely manner because the professional advocate had knowledge of the medical issue, was aware of the urgency of the situation, and knew how to access proper resources to resolve the problem. The advice to seek home health support was an unexpected but welcomed benefit that contributed to the patient's overall well-being.

What Are the Characteristics of a Good Patient Advocate?

All patient advocates, whether friends or professionals, must have excellent communication skills, sensitivity to all parties involved, and the ability to convey information with polite assertiveness. Medical knowledge and experience in the health care field are valuable assets, although they are not requirements to deliver effective patient advocacy. Listening actively, asking relevant questions, engaging patients in dialogue, and clarifying any medical concerns they may have are essential characteristics of all good patient advocates.

Whenever a family member or friend accompanies you to a medical visit, they are functioning as your advocate without being aware of it. This can be a great benefit because it helps to have another person present to hear the information being shared, to help you recall important facts about your history, and to encourage you to follow through with the doctor's recommendations.

In sum, professional patient advocates can:

o   Define and address the health care delivery challenges faced by clients.

o   Facilitate timely access to medical care.

o   Facilitate patient-doctor discussion and decision-making.

o   Ensure clarity of medical information.

o   Promote the importance of preventive health care.

o   Teach tools to promote self-advocacy.

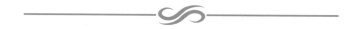

Let's take a look at how a family member who traveled across the country to give emotional support to a loved one was prompted to act as a professional advocate when she recognized that standard medical procedures were not being followed.

From Our Case Files…

J.L., a 72-year-old retired professor whose diabetes is controlled with oral medications, was hospitalized at a medical teaching hospital for a surgical procedure unrelated to the diabetes. After surgery, she received pain medication and was unable to eat, but she received fluids and nutrition through an I.V. (intravenous) line. On the second day after surgery, a nurse arrived who said, "I am here to give you your insulin." The daughter, a medical professional, immediately asked, "What is her blood sugar level?" The nurse reported, "I don't know. I was just told to give this insulin shot." The daughter replied, "My mother does not take insulin. She is controlled with oral medicines and diet." The nurse replied, "Well, I don't have her blood sugar results. So, does that mean you are refusing this medication for her?" "Yes," replied the daughter, "I am until you can tell me the results of her recent blood sugar test." *The nurse left the room and did not return. Several hours later, a different nurse came into the room and reported to the daughter that J.L.'s evening and morning blood sugar tests "were great," and therefore no insulin was required.*

What is the lesson here? Patient advocates at the bedside of hospitalized patients are invaluable. In some cases, they can prevent medical errors and even save lives. An alert and attentive bedside advocate who is willing to carefully observe the medical care being delivered and ask appropriate questions in a hospital setting can be a great asset.

In this case, J.L.'s daughter, a medical professional, was acutely aware of the standard of care and protocols around the basic treatment of a post-surgical patient with diabetes. It was therefore alarming to the daughter that such a breach of protocol could occur, especially at a teaching hospital.

There are standard clinical guidelines that medical professionals should follow at all times to protect the safety of patients. While laypeople are not usually familiar with these guidelines, most of them know the basics of blood sugar testing and the dosing of medication for diabetes management. So, in this case, patient advocacy could have been performed effectively by a peer advocate or a family member who was knowledgeable about diabetes care and treatment. In most cases, patient advocacy simply requires an attentive and caring person who is unafraid to question procedures.

Proactive or Reactive?

J.L.'s case demonstrates how family support, by necessity, can turn into patient advocacy. Usually, most of us seek patient advocates during a health crisis. This usually occurs when we are confused about our medical condition or our options, when our condition is getting worse, or when we are not getting timely responses to our questions. In many instances, the usual resources have been exhausted, and it is time to seek help. While this approach is reactive rather than proactive, it is the most common pathway to considering patient advocacy.

Patients tend to become confused when they are ill, incapacitated in any way, or out of sorts – namely, when things are just not "as they should be." We cannot stress enough the importance of having a friend or family member be aware of your medical condition. Ideally, that person should be present when you are not at your best while seeking medical care. It's comforting to have a supportive, trusted person by your side when you are faced with an urgent medical situation.

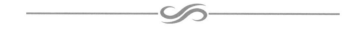

Physicians can be perceived by their patients as aloof and unempathetic. This is especially true when physicians have to inform their patients of life-altering or life-threatening diagnoses such as cancer. Imagine the near "mental paralysis" that can occur when a recurrence of cancer is diagnosed.

Professional patient advocates know that apprehension, denial, and anxiety can cloud patients' ability to make decisions about their own health, even with the best counseling and coaching by a professional patient advocate.

Let's take a look at one such case, which illustrates how confusion, fear, and distrust played a prominent role in a patient's medical decision-making.

From Our Case Files...

A.D., a 54-year-old attorney, was startled when she received a diagnosis of cancer in her left breast, because there was no history of breast cancer or any other cancer in her family. Furthermore, she felt that she had lived a very healthy lifestyle, so she questioned how this could happen to her. Eventually, she was treated with a lumpectomy (removal of cancerous tissue) and a series of radiation treatments to the breast.

Following her lumpectomy and treatment, A.D. faithfully underwent annual mammography, continued regular follow-up exams with her oncologist (cancer specialist), and was more committed than ever to pursuing a healthy lifestyle. This consistent commitment to her health increased her assurance that she was cancer-free. After 10 years of normal mammograms, however, she learned that she had cancer in her right breast, which made her skeptical, frightened, and angry. To add to A.D.'s frustration, her trusted oncologist of nine years had recently left her health plan and relocated her practice. Because of this, A.D. felt abandoned by her former oncologist and constrained by the available oncologists covered under her insurance.

When A.D. saw her new oncologist, she was advised to have a second lumpectomy and radiation treatment. However, she was not comfortable with the way the oncologist presented the information to her. Virtually "mentally paralyzed," she decided to seek the help of a physician friend.

The friend discovered that A.D. had an exceptionally trusting relationship with her previous oncologist, which was contributing to her current anxiety and skepticism. The physician friend then provided a more detailed explanation of treatment options in a supportive way. While this advocacy support was well received by A.D., she was adamant that she only wanted a lumpectomy without radiation treatment.

Five years later, living in a new location, A.D. had a third occurrence of breast cancer. She was now receiving her medical care at a world-renowned cancer center. This diagnosis was obviously another physical and emotional setback for A.D., but her ability to rely on her past experiences and the advocacy counseling she had received from her physician friend empowered her to accept the diagnosis and to confidently participate in her own medical care. A.D. tolerated the recommended treatment well, and, months later, she was confident that she had made the right decision.

What is the lesson here? Many patients are confused and stymied when faced with life-altering diagnoses such as diabetes, heart disease, or cancer. These diagnoses can cause distress and anxiety in individuals of all educational and socioeconomic levels. In our experience, the essential anchor for these patients is a stable, trusting patient-doctor relationship, which is extremely valuable when difficult decision-making is required. Building that trust contributes greatly to ensuring that patients are confident with their medical management, which can certainly improve their compliance. This cannot always be accomplished in our current health care system, in which patients sometimes change health plans and doctors every year. In this case, the physician friend provided the trust and knowledge that A.D. needed to cope with her life-altering medical condition.

A.D.'s case illustrates the importance of trust in the patient-doctor relationship and how this can be so valuable when faced with critical decisions about your health care. It also demonstrates how professional patient advocacy can be used to clarify the understanding of health issues, present factual information, and provide a safe setting for a meaningful dialogue. This type of support is often necessary to help patients who are faced with complicated medical issues and can empower the patient with the tools to confidently make the best decision.

Advocating for our children is something we know how to do. It's a natural "skill" born out of our love, commitment, and sense of obligation. Let's take a look at a case where appropriate advocacy for a child, coupled with the medical experience of the advocate resulted in a clinical outcome of the *best* kind.

From Our Case Files…

L.H., an 11-year-old male, was taken to the hospital after 10 hours of abdominal pain. He was seen in the emergency room at a pediatric center of excellence in a major metropolitan area. After waiting for almost two hours, he was seen by an ER triage nurse, who took a brief medical history and checked his vital signs. After 45 more minutes, L.H. was seen by a doctor, who examined him and ordered x-rays, lab tests, and an I.V. line. An additional four hours passed, during which time L.H. experienced continued abdominal pain and the onset of vomiting. Despite one abnormal lab test, inconclusive x-rays, and a history of 16 hours of constant abdominal pain with vomiting, the surgeon felt that it was not a "clear case" of acute appendicitis and decided that further observation was required to confirm that diagnosis.

Therefore, the surgeon decided to hand off L.H.'s care to a surgical colleague who was due to arrive *at the hospital within the hour, while he himself left the hospital to handle "another case" several miles away. The patient's mother, who had not left his side the whole time, was a medical professional who not only knew that acute appendicitis was the most likely diagnosis, but was also well versed in the time frame in which appropriate intervention should occur to avoid complications. Recognizing that an additional delay could result in a ruptured appendix, L.H.'s mother knew that her son was at risk of a potentially life-threatening condition. Therefore, she cornered the surgeon in the hallway and begged him not to hand off her son's care, but instead to take out the appendix. Within minutes, L.H.'s mother found herself helping the surgeon wheel her son to the operating floor as he was hurriedly prepared for surgery. While wheeling the gurney to the operating room, the surgeon turned to the mother and said, "I really don't think this is a case of acute appendicitis, but I will go in and remove his appendix and take a look around inside to see if I can find a reason for his abdominal pain."*

Approximately 60 minutes later, the surgeon arrived in the waiting room to report that the surgery had been successful and L.H. was doing well. The surgeon commented that he had just removed the biggest appendix he had ever seen in his professional career. L.H. was in recovery but would need to remain in the hospital for at least three days to receive intravenous antibiotics, because the surgeon could not be sure that the infection in the appendix had not leaked into the surrounding tissues. After several days, however, L.H. was discharged, had an uneventful recovery, and was able to gradually resume his usual activities.

What is the lesson here? This is an example of the value of a professional patient advocate on site in an urgent setting. In this case, the advocate just happened to be a mother who was a physician. She had the medical knowledge required to ask the appropriate questions at the appropriate time. It is noteworthy that the exchange between the treating surgeon and L.H.'s mother required polite assertiveness on the mother's part. In this case, in the end, the surgeon, the critical player, was willing to reconsider his position and move quickly to the operating room.

The need to be assertive in a medical setting is becoming more and more the norm, and the key to its success is often *how* you do it. In short, this case represents how the medical knowledge, consistent presence, and polite assertiveness of a professional patient advocate can make a difference in your best health.

Patient Advocacy: An Emerging Trend…

Patient advocacy has not only become an important consideration to assist health care consumers, but it is gaining popularity as a career choice. The success of this resource depends on effective communication, savvy navigation and appropriate advocacy. Listening to our clients and other health care consumers, we know that there are fundamental gaps in rapport that undermine the important patient-doctor relationship. This can negatively impact patients' engagement, understanding, trust, and compliance.

A recent study conducted by the Arnold P. Gold Foundation, which advocates for a respectful bedside manner, revealed the survey results of encounters of 600 people with doctors. Twelve percent said they were taken care of by doctors who didn't know their names. Twenty percent had met doctors they found "rude or condescending," and forty-seven percent said they had felt rushed by doctors. All of these impressions erode the most essential partnership in health care delivery, the patient-doctor relationship (Rozman, 2010). Failure to address the components of a healthy patient-doctor relationship will cause further frustration, mistrust, lack of compliance, medical errors and, ultimately, poor clinical outcomes. The patient advocate can mitigate much of this by understanding the challenges, pre-planning and preparing the patient for their visits, clarifying instructions, and expecting excellence in care.

With the transformation of our health care system and our aging population, the need for patient advocacy will become more and more apparent. We know the value of advocacy to the health care consumer, but until third party payers and employers recognize the economic consequences of barriers faced by patients, it is likely that this valuable resource will be limited to a select few. It is conceivable that patient advocacy could follow the same model as the employee assistance programs currently offered by many employers. Skilled patient advocates can effectively guide health care consumers through the health care maze, emphasizing the need to partner with their health care practitioner. The opportunity to witness the skills of a trained or professional advocate can empower patients to become better communicators, navigators and advocates.

As a patient, you have certain rights that should increase your confidence as you seek to improve and optimize your medical experiences through self-advocacy. These rights are outlined in several pieces of legislation. The Patient's Bill of Rights of 1997 (see Appendix II for Abridged Version) sets certain standards and expectations to ensure that patients are informed, respected, have the right to quality, emergency care, and confidentiality (HHS, 1999). The 2010 Affordable Care Act sets forth certain rights (see Appendix III for Abridged Version), designed to put patients in charge of their health care (ACA, 2010).

This Is What We Know...

There is a need for patient advocacy because:

- o Poor doctor-patient communication is the norm.

- o Medical encounters can be intimidating.

- o Our complex medical system creates barriers to access and quality care for many patients who are typically compromised at the point of entry into the health care system.

- o Patients tend to be inattentive when they are anxious and bad news is reported.

- o Limited time for doctor's appointments prevents adequate and effective interchange.

o Doctors are increasingly multitasking in order to take care of a larger volume of patients in a shorter time period.

Appropriate and successful advocacy can ensure that patients:

o Are empowered to access necessary health care when needed.

o Have the essential information required to understand their medical issues.

o Understand their treatment options.

o Demonstrate improved compliance with follow-up appointments and medications.

o Are knowledgeable and compliant with preventive health care schedules.

o Insist on receiving quality care.

As professional patient advocates, we have learned that you cannot fix everything, and we do not have the perfect solution for every case or situation. What we do know, from years of experience, is there are many factors that influence a patient's ability to become actively engaged in their health care. These include their life experiences, their preconceived notions about diseases and health, and their fear and mistrust of the medical care system. The ability of health care professionals to provide compassionate, patient-centered care will continue to be a challenge because they are overwhelmed by volumes of paper work, strict formularies, time constraints and decreasing reimbursements. Therefore, the ultimate responsibility rests with you, the patient, to take the initiative to learn about your disease, to be tenacious about asking questions, and unrelenting in your quest to achieve your *best* health.

Advocacy Tips

1. Get the right health plan for your needs.

2. Perform your due diligence to choose the right primary care doctor for you.

3. Be willing to partner with your doctor.

4. Be actively engaged during your medical encounters.

5. Bring someone with you to your doctor's appointments, if possible.

6. If there is a long wait for an appointment, ask to be considered for a cancellation.

7. Learn how to be politely assertive.

8. Be aware of signs of cultural sensitivity and competency in all health care settings.

9. Seek out resources and support groups for your specific medical condition.

10. Be knowledgeable about your medical condition and know when you need help.

11. Request that your doctors coordinate your care, especially if you have multiple medical conditions.

12. Seek a professional patient advocate if you are challenged with navigating the health care system, you are not getting your medical needs met, or if you have exhausted your resources.

13. Know your rights as a patient.

conclusion

As physicians, we know that inherent in the very nature of health care delivery is the asymmetry of knowledge: some will always have more information than others regarding a medical issue. Since it takes an average of seven to ten years to train a doctor, depending on the specialty, it is unrealistic to expect the average health care consumer to understand the causes of diseases, signs and symptoms of medical conditions, or best practices for disease management.

The 2010 Patient Protection and Affordable Care Act – long overdue – will expand accessibility to health care and preventive care for tens of thousands of Americans, but there are challenges yet to be addressed. There are some fundamental health care delivery issues that are of concern and some industry trends worthy of mention. The health care landscape continues to evolve and medical delivery models are being reinvented. One thing we can guarantee – there will be confusion!

Health insurance options will continue to change, requiring consumers to make smart, informed choices about health benefits. You should be prepared for annual increases in your monthly health insurance premiums, as well as your out-of-pocket expenses. Employer-sponsored health insurance, as we have grown to know it, is unsustainable. If you are self-employed, your choices of benefit plans are likely to be limited because of cost. Stay tuned for the expected doctor shortage of 130,000 by the year 2025. And, of course, time constraints for medical visits will not go away. This is the harsh reality of health care today and into the near future.

It is because of the transformation in health care and the uncertainty that accompanies it that you, the healthcare consumer, must continue to be involved. Be prepared to take charge and be purposeful about your medical needs in order to get the health care you deserve. Your ability to put into action the *communication, navigation,* and *advocacy* skills put forth in this book transcends economic and policy considerations. We have the highest expectations and the greatest hope that *Focus On YOUR BEST HEALTH* will provide a firm foundation, that will sustain and guide you as you seek your *best* health.

glossary

Definitions

Academic medical center: Also known as a teaching hospital, dedicated to training medical professionals and providing medical care and services to patients and communities.

Accountable Care Organization (ACO): A model of health care delivery and medical management that promotes improved coordination of patient care and quality of care in an effort to control health care costs.

Acronym: An abbreviation made up of the initial letter of a phrase or term. Example: Chief Medical Officer (CMO).

Activities of Daily Living (ADL): Daily personal care routines such as bathing, dressing, meal preparation and other routine activities.

Adverse reaction: Any unexpected or unwanted effect from medications, food, or procedures.

Affordable Care Act (ACA): The federal health care law passed by Congress and signed into law by President Obama on March 23, 2010. It is intended to decrease the number of uninsured Americans and as well as the overall cost of health care (www.healthcare.gov).

Anterior Cruciate Ligament (ACL): One of four ligaments of the knee joint. This ligament controls the back and forth motion of your knee and is commonly injured in athletes.

Aspiration: The removal of body fluids or substances from body cavities using suction, typically with a needle/syringe.

Bed-side Manner: A term describing how a healthcare professional builds rapport, demonstrates compassion, and effectively communicates with patients.

Biopsy: A procedure used to obtain a sample of tissue for purposes of microscopic examination.

Blood culture: A laboratory test performed on a blood sample, used to detect the presence of bacteria or other organisms within the blood stream.

Board Certification: The successful completion of a process of standardized testing, confirming a doctor's mastery of a particular area of medicine in a specialty and/or subspecialty.

Burn-out: A condition characterized by emotional exhaustion which can affect physical health, emotional well-being, performance, and job productivity.

Caesarean section: A surgical procedure that involves making an incision in the abdomen and the uterus to deliver a baby.

Cardiopulmonary (CP): Term that refers to involvement of the heart and the lungs.

Catheterization: A medical procedure that involves passing a small tube through a body organ, vessel or chamber, usually with radiologic visualization.

Certified language interpreter: An individual who has passed a standardized certification examination, confirming proficiency in language translation.

Chronic obstructive pulmonary disease (COPD): Chronic lung diseases that include chronic bronchitis and emphysema.

Clinical outcome: The change in the medical condition of a patient following a medical treatment or intervention.

Colonoscopy: A medical procedure that involves the introduction of a flexible tube into the rectum, allowing visualization of the colon (large intestine). This test is considered the gold standard for colon cancer screening.

Computerized tomography (CT/Cat scan): A body imaging technique that uses x-rays to get detail pictures of tissues and organs of the body.

Concierge medicine: A medical practice model dedicated to personalized care. The health care consumer can engage a primary care doctor and pay an annual retainer fee for services rendered.

Cultural literacy: Knowledge of the history, values, and perspectives of different cultural groups that contribute to the understanding of population groups other than your own.

Cultural sensitivity: "The knowledge and interpersonal skills that allow providers to understand, appreciate, and work with individuals from cultures other than their own. It involves an awareness and acceptance of cultural differences, self awareness, knowledge of a patient's culture, and adaptation of skills." (Fleming M, Towey K., AMA 2001)

Cultural competency: "Competency is the capacity to function effectively as an individual and an organization within the context of the cultural beliefs, behaviors, and needs presented by consumers and their communities." (Adapted from Cross, 1989)

Cystoscopy: A medical procedure performed by introducing a scope into the urethra (a tube through which urine is discharged from the kidney) that allows visualization of the inside lining of the structures of the urinary tract and the bladder.

Defensive medicine: The practice of doctors ordering diagnostic medical testing or treatments not for the sole benefit to the patient, but because of the threat of medical liability.

Do Not Resuscitate (DNR): A legal order written in the hospital or on a legal form as a directive to respect the wishes of a patient not to undergo CPR (cardio pulmonary resuscitation) or advanced cardiac life support if they experience respiratory arrest (stop breathing) or if their heart stops beating.

Echocardiogram: A diagnostic procedure that uses sound waves to create a picture of the heart to detect abnormalities of the chambers, valves, blood flow, and heart function.

Endoscope: A flexible or rigid tube equipped with a light source used to visualize the interior of body organs.

Endoscopy: A medical procedure that allows for visualization of body organs, utilizing a special instrument, an endoscope.

End Stage Renal Disease (ESRD): The last stage of chronic kidney disease that requires either dialysis or kidney transplant in order for the patient to stay alive.

Fellow: A term used to refer to an individual who has completed a medical residency and is now engaged in additional sub-specialty training, usually 1-3 years.

Gen X-ers: A segment of the population born between the early 1960s and early 1980s.

Gen Y-ers: A segment of the population born between the late 1970s and early 2000s, also referred to as the millennial generation.

Geriatrics: A subspecialty of internal medicine and family medicine that focuses on the health care of the elderly.

Gurney: A trolley or stretcher used to transport patients.

"Hand-off": The process of transferring the responsibility for care of a patient from one medical care provider to another.

Health literacy: "The degree to which individuals have the capacity to obtain, process, and understand basic health information and services needed to make appropriate health decisions." (Healthy People 2012)

Health Maintenance Organization (HMO): A health insurance plan made up of an alliance of medical professionals, allied health workers, and facilities contracted with insurance companies to provide services at an agreed upon fixed price.

Hemodialysis: A medical procedure that allows for the removal of waste products from the body such as urea or creatinine, when the kidneys fail and are unable to function.

Holistic health: Defined by the American Holistic Association as "the conscious pursuit of the highest level of functioning and balance of the physical, environmental, mental, emotional, social and spiritual aspects of human experience, resulting in a dynamic state of being fully alive."

Hospitalist: A doctor who is exclusively hospital -based and cares for you when you are in the hospital.

July effect: A phenomenon that occurs in July of every year when more experienced doctors -in-training in teaching hospitals are replaced by newly minted medical school graduates.

Local medical society: A professional organization of physicians that supports doctors by assisting them in communicating and collaborating with their peers and the local medical community to improve quality of care for patients.

Mammogram: A diagnostic and screening test for breast cancer that uses low energy x-rays.

Managed care: Healthcare plans or systems designed to control medical costs by contracting with a network of specific providers and requiring pre-authorization for visits to specialist and other allied health professionals. The medical care can be delivered by doctors and other medical professionals who are affiliated with HMO or PPO organizations.

Medical formulary: A list of drugs approved by and paid for by health plans or other health care payers based on a contracted financial arrangement with the supplier.

Medical Home: A model of health care delivery and medical management in a patient-centered environment, designed to promote more effective delivery of primary care medicine by improving patient safety, efficiency and quality of care.

Medical jargon: The language of medicine that includes acronyms, medical terminology, and abbreviations.

Medical narrative: A patient's medical story that provides pertinent information that will enhance the patient-doctor encounter and make the visit most relevant.

Magnetic Resonance Imaging (MRI): A body scanning technique that uses a magnetic field and radio waves to make pictures of organs and structures inside the body. It does not use radiation like traditional x-rays or CT scans.

Network: A group of doctors, hospitals, ancillary healthcare professionals, and pharmacies enrolled in health plans as health care providers to deliver medical services to plan members.

Nurse practitioner (NP): A nurse with a graduate degree in advanced practice nursing. Many NPs function as independent providers of medical care.

Over-the-counter (OTC): Over-the-counter medicines are drugs you can buy without a prescription.

Paratransit: A type of passenger transportation that provides services to the elderly and to patients with disabilities.

Patient-centered health care: Health care that places patients as the central focus, including them and their family members as active participants in clinical decision-making. The delivery of patient-centered care should have at its core acknowledgment and consideration of the patient's traditions, culture, preferences, and values.

Patient-controlled analgesic (PCA): A method by which patients self-deliver intravenous narcotic pain medication.

Perfect storm: A term used to describe an untoward event resulting from a combination of occurrences which if considered singularly would not be considered noteworthy.

Phlebotomist: A technician trained in collecting blood samples for diagnostic testing and blood donations.

Physician assistant (PA): A healthcare professional trained to practice medicine under the supervision of a physician. Many PAs function as independent providers of medical care.

Physician extender: A trained health care professional who is not a physician, but who performs medical activities that are usually performed by a physician, and can include nurse practitioners and physician assistants.

Positron emission tomography scan (PET scan): A type of body imaging test that uses a small dose of radioactive material ('tracer') injected into the arm which travels to different organs and helps doctors visualize how the organs and tissues of your body are functioning.

PPO (preferred provider organization): A managed care plan that has a panel of preferred providers contracted with insurance companies to provide medical services to patients for an agreed upon price. These plans allow more flexibility with regard to selection of primary care physicians and specialists than health maintenance organizations.

Prior authorization (pre-authorization): A method of controlling costs. In health care this is done by requiring pre-approval of some visits and diagnostic testing.

Prognostic: Prediction of the future outcome of a disease or a condition.

Resident: A medical school graduate engaged in post-graduate medical training in special branches of medicine.

Skilled nursing facility: An in-patient health care facility where patients receive non-acute care, prescribed nursing care and other therapies.

Specialty: A branch of medicine or surgery specialization such as pediatrics or urology.

Subspecialty: A specific field of expertise within the specialty branch of medicine or surgery such as cardiology.

Specialty medical society: An organization such as the American Academy of Dermatology or the American College of Cardiology that provides a platform for doctors of that specialty to share ideas and best practices with the ultimate goal of improving patient care.

Teach-back: A communication technique used to confirm that the patient understands what they need to know about their medical condition based on the doctor's explanation.

Teaching hospital: A hospital, typically closely associated with a medical school, dedicated to providing clinical education and training to future doctors, existing medical staff, nurses, and other health care professionals.

Traditional health insurance plan: This is the fee-for-service insurance model where doctors are paid for each service rendered and bills are submitted to insurers (insurance companies) for payment.

Triage nurse: A health care team member who makes initial assessments of patients/medical problems to determine acuity.

Ultrasound: A diagnostic test that uses sound waves to determine the status of body organs and tissues.

Your Personal Health Record (YPHR): A paper version of a personal health record that includes your pertinent medical information including past medical history, family history, medical interventions (surgeries), medications, immunizations, allergies, recent diagnostic tests, dates of routine preventive health tests and procedures, previous hospitalizations/surgeries, emergency contact information, health insurance information, and contact information for your primary care doctor.

Commonly Used Abbreviations/Acronyms

ACL - Anterior cruciate ligament

BE - Barium enema

BKA - Below the knee amputation

BMI - Body mass index

BP - Blood pressure

CT/CAT scan - Computerized axial tomography scan

CBC - Complete blood count

COPD - Chronic obstructive pulmonary disease

CP - Cardiopulmonary

DDX - Differential diagnosis

DM - Diabetes mellitus

DNR - Do not resuscitate

ESRD - End stage renal disease

HBP - High blood pressure

I.V. - Intravenous

KCL - Potassium chloride

MRI - Magnetic Resonance Imaging

MVP - Mitral valve prolapse

PET Scan - Positron Emission Tomography scan

RA - Rheumatoid arthritis

UTI - Urinary tract infection

p.r.n. - as needed

q.d. - once a day

q.h.s. - every night at bedtime

t.i.d. - three times a day

Commonly Used Medical Jargon/The Language of Medicine

Aneurysm: An abnormal widening or ballooning of a portion of an artery due to weakness in the wall of the blood vessel.

Anuric: Not producing urine.

Bibasilar: Abnormal breath sounds heard at the base of both lungs, often noted with pneumonia.

Cardiopulmonary: Involving the cardia (heart) and pulmonary (lungs).

Cerebrovascular accident: A stroke caused by blockage of an artery in the brain, or a blood clot to the brain from the heart or carotid (neck) artery, or hemorrhage (bleeding) into the brain.

Curettage: The removal of tissue or growths from a body cavity, such as the uterus, by scraping with a curette (instrument).

Dilation: To enlarge or expand an organ or vessel as in the treatment of esophageal stricture (partial closure of the esophagus) or heart vessel disease. This term is also used to describe the naturally occurring expansion of the cervix during childbirth.

Dyscrasia: A nonspecific term that refers to any disease or disorder, but it usually refers to blood diseases.

Dysplasia: An abnormal development or growth of tissues, organs, or cells.

Encephalopathy: A nonspecific term describing a syndrome affecting the brain. It typically refers to involvement of large parts of the brain (or the whole organ).

Edema: An abnormal accumulation of fluid beneath the skin or in one or more cavities of the body that produces swelling. Edema was formerly known as dropsy or hydropsy. Edema happens most often in the feet, ankles, and legs.

Myopathy: A muscular disease affecting the muscle fibers making them weak.

Prolapse: This term literally means "to fall out of place." It is usually used to describe conditions where organs have loss their normal structure and integrity.

Retinal: An adjective used to describe conditions related to the retina as in retinal detachment. The retina is the light-sensitive tissue lining the inner surface of the eye.

Stat: An abbreviation that means "immediately" and used in communication of medical orders.

Stenosis: An abnormal narrowing in a blood vessel or other tubular organ or structure such as the aorta.

Vitals: An even shorter abbreviation for vital signs used in medicine to include blood pressure, body temperature, heart rate, and respiratory (breathing) rate.

appendix I

Your Personal Health Record

Your Personal Health Record

Family History _____

_____

_____

_____

Health Care Practitioner_____

MD, NP, PA_____

Phone #_____

Preferred Hospital_____

Emergency Contact_____

Notes _____

_____

_____

_____

_____

Name _____

Health Insurance_____

   Group#_____

Allergies_____

_____

Medical Conditions _____

_____

_____

_____

Medications_____

_____

Previous Hospitalization/Surgeries_____

_____

_____

Your Personal Health Contract

Age 20
- Primary Care Physician Exam with Labs Annually
- Pap Smear with HPV Screen at age 21
- Immunizations - TB Screening, Tdap, HPV, Meningiococcal (partial listing)
- Testicular Exam (Males Only)
- HIV Testing

Age 30
- Primary Care Physician Exam with Labs, Pap with HPV Annually
- Immunizations - TB Screening, Tdap, Flu (partial listing)
- HIV Testing

Age 40
- Primary Care Physician Exam with Labs, Pap with HPV Annually
- Immunizations - TB Screening, Tdap, Flu (partial listing)
- PSA with Digital Rectal Exam Annually (Males Only)
- Mammogram Annually (if positive family history check with your health care practitioner)
- HIV Testing

Age 50
- Primary Care Physician Exam with Labs Annually
- Immunizations - TB Screening, Tdap, Flu (partial listing)
- Sigmoidoscopy/Colonoscopy Every 5-10 years
- Mammogram Annually
- HIV Testing

Age 60

- Primary Care Physician Exam with Labs (PSA) and Pap, and Mammogram Annually
- Immunizations - TB Screening, Tdap, Pneumovac, Herpes Zoster, Flu
- Osteoporosis (Bone Density Screening)
- Sigmoidoscopy/Colonoscopy Every 5-10 years
- Abdominal Aneurysm Screening (age 65)
- HIV Testing

My Personal Health Pledge

At the designated age and the appropriate time interval I, _____, pledge to follow through with the recommended preventive health care measures/screening.

Signature_____

Date_____

www.nandsconsulting.com

© 2013 Newell and Spriggs Consulting, LLC

appendix II

Patient's Bill of Rights 1997-1998

Patient's Bill of Rights (1997-1998)

Objectives

o   To strengthen consumer confidence by assuring the health care system is fair and responsive to consumers' needs, provides consumers with credible and effective mechanisms to address their concerns, and encourages consumers to take an active role in improving and assuring their health.

o   To reaffirm the importance of a strong relationship between patients and their health care professionals.

o   To reaffirm the critical role consumers play in safeguarding their own health by establishing both rights and responsibilities for all participants in improving health status.

Rights and Responsibilities

I. Information Disclosure

Patients have the right to receive accurate, easily understood information to help them make informed decisions about their health plans, professionals and facilities.

II. Choice of Providers and Plans

Consumers have the right to a choice of health care providers that is sufficient to ensure access to appropriate high-quality health care.

III. Access to Emergency Services

Consumers have the right to access emergency health care services when and where the need arises.

IV. Participation in Treatment Decisions

Consumers have the right and responsibility to fully participate in all decisions related to their health care.

V. Respect and Nondiscrimination

Consumers have the right to considerate, respectful care from all members of the health care system at all times and under all circumstances. An environment of mutual respect is essential to maintain a quality health care system.

VI. Confidentiality of Health Information

Consumers have the right to communicate with health care providers in confidence and to have the confidentiality of their individually identifiable health care information protected. Consumers also have the right to review and copy their own medical records and request amendments to their records.

VII. Complaints and Appeals

All consumers have the right to a fair and efficient process for resolving differences with their health plans, health care providers, and the institutions that serve them, including a rigorous system of internal review and an independent system of external review.

VIII. Consumer Responsibilities

In a health care system that protects consumers' rights, it is reasonable to expect and encourage consumers to assume reasonable responsibilities. Greater individual involvement by consumers in their care increases the likelihood of achieving the best outcomes and helps support a quality improvement, cost-conscious environment.

Complete Details: http://www.opm.gov/healthcare-insurance/healthcare/consumer-protections/#url=Bill-of-Rights

appendix III

Patient's Bill of Rights
Patient Protection and Affordable Care Act of 2010

Patient's Bill of Rights

The Affordable Care Act puts consumers back in charge of their health care. Under the law, a new "Patient's Bill of Rights" gives the American people the stability and flexibility they need to make informed choices about their health.

o   Provides Coverage to Americans with Pre-existing Conditions

o   Protects Your Choice of Doctors

o   Keeps Young Adults Covered on Parent's health insurance until Age 26

o   Ends Lifetime Limits on Coverage

o   Ends Pre-Existing Condition Exclusions for Children

o   Ends Arbitrary Withdrawals of Insurance Coverage

o   Reviews Health Insurance Premium Increases Imposed by Insurance Companies

o   Helps You Get the Most from Your Premium Dollars

o   Restricts Annual Dollar Limits on Coverage

o   Removes Insurance Company Barriers to Emergency Services o   Covers Preventive Care at No Cost to You

o   Guarantees Your Right to Appeal

Complete Details: http://www.healthcare.gov/law/features/
rights/bill-of-rights/index.html

references

References

American Academy of Private Physicians (AAPP); (2000), http://www.aapp.org/

American Holistic Medical Association (AHMA), (2012) http://www.holisticmedicine.org.

American Medical Association (AMA), (2013) "Informed Consent," http://ama-assn.org/ama/pub/physician-resources/legal-topics/patient-physician-relationship-topics/informed-consent.page.

American Telemedicine Association (ATA), (2012) "What is Telemedicine?" www.americantelemed.org/learn.

Anderson G., Horvath J., "The growing burden of chronic disease in America." Public Health Reports 2004;119: 263-70.

Anderson, Laurie, M., et al. Cultural Competent Healthcare Systems: A Systematic Review. *Am J Prev Med* 2003:24 (3S).

Ask Me 3™, http://www.npsf.org/for-healthcare-professionals/programs/ask-me-3, 2011.

Baker, Sharon, "Hospitalists No Longer Novel," *MANAGED CARE*, February 2006. http://www.managedcaremag.com/archives/0602/0602.hospitalists.html

California Healthline, "Health Reform Law Could Worsen Doctor Shortage, Experts Say," (2012) http://www.californiahealthline.org/articles/2012/7/30/health-reform-law-could-worsen-doctor-shortage-experts-say.aspx.

Centers for Disease Control, Diabetes Research and Statistics, Last updated February 16, 2012. http://www.cdc.gov/diabetes/consumer/research.htm.

Diversity Council (2008), "Cross-Cultural Communication: Translating Nonverbal Cues," 2008; www.diversitycouncil.org/toolkit/Resources_TipSheet_NonverbalCrossCulturalCommunication. pdf.

Gogoi, P., "Steering Patients Through the System: Quantum Health Points to the Best Care-and Saves Employers Big Bucks," *Businessweek*, February 27, 2006.

Harris, Gardiner, "New for Aspiring Doctors, The People Skills Test," *The New York Times*, 7.10.11.

Hospital Physician Partners (HPPartners), "The Growth of Hospitalists and Hospitalist Jobs," July 26, 2011, http://www.hppartners.com/blog/the-growth-of-hospitalists-and-hospitalist-jobs.

Jenks, Stephen, Williams, Mark, Coleman, Eric, "Rehospitalizations among Patients in the Medicare Fee-for-Service Program," *N Engl J Me*, 2009; 360:1418-1428.

Johnson, Dirk, "A $42 Million Gift Aims at Improving Bedside Manner," *The New York Times*, 9.22.11.

Krupa, Carolyne, "New residents linked to July medication errors." *Journal of General Internal Medicine.* June 21, 2012. http://www.ama-assn.org/amednews/2010/06/21/prsb0621.htm.

Maizes, Victoria, David Rakel, Catherine Niemiec. Integrative Medicine and Patient-Centered Care, Commissioned for the IOM Summit on Integrative Medicine and the Health of the Public, February, 2009.

Morasch, Laura Johnson, "I Hear You But I Don't Understand You!": Medical Jargon & Clear Communication, Molina Healthcare and California Academy of Family Physicians (2005).

National Association of Insurance Commissioners (NAIC), "Boomers in the Sandwich Generation Face Complex Insurance Decisions," http://www.naic.org/ Releases/2012)_docs/boomers_insurance_decisions.htm.

National Center on Senior Transportation (NCST); (2012), www.seniortransportation.net.

NYU Macy Initiative on Health Communication (2001), NYU Medical School. http://nyumacy.med.nyu.edu/index. html.

Phillips D.P., Barker, G.E., "A July spike in fatal medication errors: a possible effect of new medical residents." *J Gen Intern Med*. Aug; 25 (8):774-9. Epub 2010 May 29.

Rozman, Katherine, "The Power of Compassion." April 13, 2010, http://online.wsj.com/article/SB100014240527023036 01504575154213442316070.html.

Runy, Lee Ann. "Patient Handoffs: The Pitfalls and Solutions of Transferring Patients Safely for One Caregiver to Another." *Hospital & Health Networks*, accessed May 10, 2012.www. hhnmag.com/hhnmag/gateFold/PDF/05_2008/5.08_hhn_ gate.pdf.

Shanafelt, Tait MD, Boone, Sonja, MD, Tan, Litjen, PhD, et al, "Burnout and Satisfaction With Work-Life Balance Among US Physicians Relative to the General Population," *Arch Intern Med.* August 20, 2012.

Stewart, M.A., "Effective physician - patient communication and health outcomes: a review," *CMAJ. JAMC*, 1995; 152 (9):1423-1433.

The Affordable Care Act (ACA), 3 March 2010, "The Health Care Law and You," http://www.healthcare.gov/law/ index.html.

The Affordable Care Act (ACA) 2010, Patient's Bill of Rights, http://www.healthcare.gov/law/features/rights/bill-of-rights/index.html.

Thiedke, C. Carolyn MD. "What Do We Really Know About

Patient Satisfaction?" *Family Practice Management*, 14 Jan 2007; 14:(1):33-36.

The Institute of Medicine, "To Err is Human: Building a Safer Health System," www.iom.edu/~/media/Files/ReportFiles/1999/To-Err-is-Human/To Err is Human 1999 report brief. pdf.

Tucker, Carolyn M., et al. "Patient-Centered Culturally Sensitive Health Care: Model Testing and Refinement," Health Psychology, 2011, May 30 (3):342-50, Psycnet.apa.org/journals/hea/30/3/3421.

Tu Ha T., Lauer, Johanna, "Word of Mouth and Physician Referrals Still Drive Health Care Provider Choice," (2008) HSC Research Brief #9,www.hschange.com/CONTENT/10281.

U.S. Department of Education; Office of Civil Rights, Rehabilitation Act of 1973, www2.ed.gov/about/offices/list/ocr/docs/edlite-August 2010.

U.S. Department of Health and Human Services (HHS), HHS.GovARCHIVE, April 12, 1999, http://archive.hhs.

gov/news/press/1999pres/990412.html.

Yach D, Hawkes C., Gould C.L., Hofman, K.J., "The global burden of chronic diseases: overcoming impediments to prevention and control." *JAMA*. 2004; 291:2616-22.

Young, John Q. MD, MPP; Ranji, Sumant R., MD; Wachter, Robert M. MD, etal.,"July Effect: Impact of the Academic Year-End Changeover on Patient Outcomes: A Systematic Review." An Intern Med. 6 September 2011; 155 (5): 309-315.

acknowledgments

From concept to completion of this book, we have been fortunate to have the encouragement and support of family members, colleagues, mentors and friends. First, we want to offer a special thank you to Price Cobbs, M.D. for his unwavering guidance and encouragement from the very beginning of our journey; to Wendy Posner, who is a clear communicator and realist when it comes to promotional endeavors; to Donna Tate of Gra De Ent Design, our creative point person, and to Jacqui Love Thornell for her editorial assistance. Also, we would like to extend a very special thank you to Toni Martin, M.D., who has been extraordinary in her response to every SOS we dispatched and who has served as a superb sounding board. We would like to thank Tracie Payne of CUSH Communications, Inc. for her expert guidance and patience as we prepared this book for publication. We must acknowledge Mr. Cleo Streets, Mr. Phillip Harris, Barbara Davis Irving, Esq. Robert L. Harris, Esq., Barbara Parker, Esq., Professor Virginia K. Newell, and Charles M. Cannady, Ph.D. for their steadfast understanding and patience, especially during the moments when we were consumed with the stresses that accompany deadlines, writer's block, work overloads, doubts, and multiple re-writes. Finally, we could not have completed this project without the clients, family members and friends who allowed us to share their medical experiences that not only became the catalyst for this book, but which gave us the ingredients to deliver authentic representations of consumers' involvement with our health care system. We are humbled by and grateful to you all.

about the authors

Glenda F. Newell, M.D., a board certified physician in Internal Medicine, is a media spokesperson on new advances in medicine and controversial medical issues which has made her a valued medical expert. Through her exceptional talents, she has engaged faith-based, professional and medical audiences about tough, complicated health topics. Having served as a local health commissioner and a leader of local and regional medical societies, she is a sought after speaker for youth groups, non-profit organizations that mentor pre-med and medical students, as well as professional organizations.

Dr. Newell is a leading medical consultant in healthcare settings, inclusive of ambulatory teaching clinics. She has served as Medical Director of Primary Care Services for a leading, cutting-edge non-profit medical organization, and has further been recognized for her work as chair of health and wellness for the Links, Incorporated, a major international philanthropic organization.

A native of North Carolina, a graduate of Miss Porter's School, Tufts University and the University of Cincinnati School of Medicine, she has received certification in Physician Leadership in Managing Ambulatory Care from the Harvard School of Public Health.

Brenda B. Spriggs, M.D. MPH MBA, a recognized expert in her chosen specialty, served as chief of rheumatology at Children's Hospital, San Francisco, and has been an active member of the clinical faculty at the University of California, San Francisco, where she was conferred the status of Clinical Professor Emerita in 2006.

Dr. Spriggs' commitment to improving access to quality medical care goes beyond her professional clinical career. She is the co-founder of Newell & Spriggs Consulting, LLC, a healthcare company dedicated to meeting the evolving needs of consumers in the healthcare arena.

Dr. Spriggs has served as a board director of the Women's Foundation of California and is a founding director of One PacificCoast Bank, FSB, organizations that are successfully addressing health, social and economic injustices that affect the most vulnerable in our communities – causes about which she is most passionate.

A graduate of Fisk University and Meharry Medical College, she received her rheumatology training as a N.I.H. fellow at the University of California, San Francisco. She is a Fellow of the American College of Physicians and the American College of Rheumatology. She received her M.P.H. for Healthcare Executives at UCLA and her M.B.A. at the Peter F. Drucker and Masatoshi Ito Graduate School of Management, Claremont Graduate University.